REFLEXOLOGY:

ART, SCIENCE & HISTORY

BY CHRISTINE ISSEL

New Frontier Publishing
P.O. Box 245855, Sacramento, CA 95824

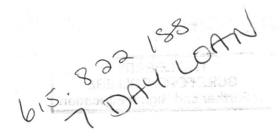

Book design and layout by David S. Issel.

ISBN: 0-9625448-2-5

First Printing: February 1990
Revised and Expanded: December 1990
Revised and Expanded: April 1993

10 9 8 7 6 5 4 3 2 1

*The information in this book is not intended
as a substitute for medical care. If you have
a health problem, consult a medical
professional.*

This book is available at a special discount
when ordered in bulk quantities. Contact
New Frontier Publishing P.O. Box 245855,
Sacramento, CA 95824.

WITHDRAWN

CONTENTS

FOREWORD

*T*hese are indeed most interesting times for Reflexology. Christine Issel has created a masterpiece of educational material that will assist in the development of our profession.

Reflexology: Art, Science & History is a shining example of the rich history that transverses many civilizations. As you will read, reflexology has its origins dating back to ancient cultures where the body was treated as a whole and the feet offered vital clues to the client's state of health.

Christine takes the reader on an exciting journey into the world of reflexology. No stone has been left unturned in her relentless search to bring as much information to the reader about reflexology. She presents all this exciting information in a very readable and interesting format and goes on to offer charts for a full comprehension of the topic. Her thorough research is of the highest standard. I enthusias-tically recommend this text to all my students in that they will have a solid foundation of knowledge.

Christine Issel has performed one of the most exceptional tasks: to gather our history on the one hand, and create it on another. Her work here will be recorded in future history as a true masterpiece. Chris's leadership and work to move reflexology into a profession through the formation of organizations and conferences which have brought reflexologists around the world together for the first time is also history in the making.

In the words of Victor Hugo, "There is one thing stronger than all the armies in the world, and that is an idea whose time has come." The time for Reflexology has come and how fortu-nate are we to have this text and the author as a guide.

Sandi Rogers
April 1993
Melbourne

THANKS...

*N*o man is an island, and no author writes a book alone. I would like to publicly acknowledge and thank those who have contributed to this work.

Foremost, to my son, David Issel, without whose valuable computer expertise this book would have remained, at most, but a manuscript.

My thanks also go to Walt Gosting and Norman Secker for their editorial assistance, constructive criticism and good ideas. Their help made this a better book than it would have otherwise been.

I am indebted to David Allan, Mildred Carter, Larry Clemmons, Bill Flocco, Walt Gosting, Jim Ingram, Harvey Lampell, Betty Lonning, George Parnell, May Post, Mrs. L.S. Relleen, Joel Swartz, Josephine Tan, Mary Lou Vanderlaan, and other reflexologists who shared their knowledge freely so that it could be recorded for the benefit of us all.

Some people added a unique dimension to this work and a special recognition is in order for them. This includes Kevin and Barbara Kunz for their encouragement of the project and a willing ear as I worked through the research material. Also to Sandi Rogers who acts as a catalyst to my mind, inspiring me to look at reflexology from new points of view. And to Dr. Simon Wikler for his legacy to reflexology, which Sandi was able to grasp.

Next, my gratitude goes to Sally and Jim Ingram for their hospitality, and to Jim for his help with some of my research interviews.

To my translators: Richard Lewis for his original German translation of Cornelius' book, Fabrice Marion for the translation of a French treatise, and Diamela Wetzl for translating the Spanish charts. Thank you all.

Also thanks to Paul Toan for contributing the Chinese hand charts which I had translated, and his acupuncture knowledge. And to Ramiro Roman who brought *Masaje Zonal En Los Pies* to my attention.

Heartfelt thanks to Sue Langer and her Indian contacts for the translation of the painting on the cover.

To the Best Care Company of Tokyo, Japan who expanded my horizions and stimulated me to include, in the second printing, the Eastern history; I am most grateful.

For the use of their photographs I owe a word of thanks to Toni Wilbanks, Josephine Tan and David Issel.

To Josephine Whipple who first introduced me to the benefits of reflexology and what it can achieve, I owe a special debt of gratitude.

I am much obliged to Janie Stauduhar, my first client whose body demonstrated what reflexology can accomplish.

Also to Lourdes Rabago who asked me to develop a curriculum and thus began my research.

Thank you Dwight Byers of the International Institute of Reflexology for teaching me the Original Ingham method of reflexology in 1976. This began a career which has made it possible for me to help so many people.

To the authors who have gone before me, thank you for leaving a trail for me to follow. Your work has been an inspiration to me.

And last, but not least to my husband Richard and our other three children, Lena, April and Jason who all made sacrifices so that I could conduct my research and struggle with writing the text.

I appreciate the contributions of those listed above, and you my reader. Thank you.

DEDICATION

*T*his book is dedicated to reflexologists everywhere: May the information within these pages add to your appreciation of our profession.

INTRODUCTION

"Cornelius was probably the first to apply massage to 'reflex zones' even though he was apparently unfamiliar with the work of Henry Head."

*T*hat sentence jumped off the page at me when I first read it in the Spring of 1986 as I was preparing a curriculum in reflexology for a massage school. As a reflexologist one of the concepts first taught is that, historically, reflexology developed from zone therapy. When I read the words "Head zones" I had to know if that referred to zones as reflexologists commonly referred to them or something else. What does Head have to do with reflex zones I wondered? Who would have thought that to answer that simple question would be like putting together the pieces of a puzzle? Or that it would occupy three years of my life. Or that I would spend time at Stanford University researching amongst one hundred year old, dusty and decaying medical journals and treatises. Or that the search for an answer would entail a trip to a gold rush town of the 1850's and would result in the gathering of 36" of xeroxed materials. Surely not me, but the quest had begun. One answer found led to many more questions which in turn led to more research via world-wide data banks, rare book publishers and countless personal interviews, all of which has culminated in this work.

Many discoveries, in any kind of research, be it scientific or historical, are the result of accidents. Research is often serendipity—full of unexpected surprises. Facts just drop into the researcher's lap. For instance, while I was helping my daughter with a college psychology paper I ran across the origin of the word "reflexology" in one of the reference books she was using.

In doing research one quickly realizes all discoveries come down from someone else's discoveries, which happen because someone before them discovered something else. There is a trail, sometimes faint and often filled with gaps, but nonetheless a trail to follow. Ideas or thoughts do not just appear out of thin air. As I soon discovered, this is true with the story of reflexology. American physician William Fitzgerald, credited for being the father of zone therapy, is not the beginning and end to the chronicle of zone therapy or reflexology as has previously been written. The history and scientific basis of reflexology actually links Russia, the United States, England and Germany together. It includes pioneering work by medical doctors, knighted physicians, and Nobel Prize winners.

Another aspect to consider regarding the history of reflexology is that the practice of foot work appears in a variety of cultures throughout history in different ages, and in sites far removed from each other. As Barbara and Kevin Kunz theorize in their publication *Reflexions*, reflexology may well be an archetypal form of foot work found everywhere in the world. Is it of Western or Oriental origin? Does that matter? I believe it is an archetypal therapy, and without apologies, I have intentionally narrowed my field of research to neglected Western sources, although a few Eastern systems will be touched upon from time to time.

The reader will note there is a discrepancy between the history contained here and that found in *Reflex Zone Therapy of the Feet* by Hanne Marquardt which was published in Germany in 1974. She took her historical material largely from the work of H.B. Bressler, who had published his book *Zone Therapy* in 1956. Unfortunately, probably due to an error in translation, Marquardt's history is incorrect, and therefore subsequent authors who have used Marquardt as a source are also incorrect.

There's a saying in publishing that a book is obsolete once it reaches print. This is true. Our knowledge on any subject is constantly changing and being revised as new knowledge is uncovered. This work is a first publishing draft on the art, science and history of reflexology. It is certainly not to be viewed as a "complete" work or the "last" word on the subject. Actually, it is meant to be a point of departure to spur readers on to their own research. I accept that it will be necessary to modify some details and explanations as our scientific and historical knowledge expands. Therefore, bringing to my attention, through the publisher, any verifiable historical information that has been omitted will be welcomed and appreciated. The same applies to other theories on the scientific basis of reflexology, as well as thoughts about the art of reflexology. Contributions to further expand Chapters 8 and 9 will be gratefully accepted.

Reflexology: Art, Science and History is simply my attempt to share what I have uncovered in the hope it provides the reader a greater appreciation of his art. You are free to use any material in this book. My only request is that you give proper credit to sources when doing so. Thank you.

Christine Issel
November 1989
Sacramento

SECTION I

The
History of
Reflexology

CHAPTER 1

ANCIENT HISTORY
2,500 B.C. - 1850 A.D.

*I*n 1913, English anthropologist, medical doctor and researcher W.H.R. Rivers wrote:

"The outstanding problem of today (in medical research) is to determine how far similar practices in different parts of the world have arisen independently and how far they are the outcome of transmission from people to people."[1]

The challenge today is still the same, particularly in researching the origins of reflexology. Barbara and Kevin Kunz of Albuquerque, founders of *Reflexions, The Journal of the Reflexology Research Project*, theorize reflexology may well be an archetypal form of therapy found everywhere in the world.[2] This concept seems to be true. No one culture can claim to have "discovered" reflexology because different forms of working on the feet to effect health have been used by people all over the world since the beginning of time. This practice appears in diverse cultures throughout history in different ages and in sites far removed from each other. It is evident that the relationship between the feet and the internal organs of the body has been recognized by civilizations back beyond recorded history.

At present, not enough is known to determine with certainty the exact history of reflexology. The story is filled with gaps, but it has been established that cultures including those in India, Japan, China, and Europe have left traces of foot work. Since no early written record has yet been discovered, the earliest evidence of the practice of reflexology is found in the form of pictures or statues.

THE EGYPTIANS

The oldest documentation that could be interpreted as depicting the use of reflexology is found in Egypt. Dr. Joe Shelby Riley makes the statement, "The science (reflexology) you are here going into, is as old as Egypt. It was known to the ancient Egyptians and Grecians, and to ancient Arabia..."[3] Ed and Ellen Case of Los Angeles, while on a tour of Egypt with Dr. Gwendolyn Raines, were the first, in 1979, to discover concrete proof of this. The Cases brought back an ancient Egyptian papyrus scene depicting medical practitioners treating the hands and feet of their patients in 2,500 B.C.

The Egyptians contributed greatly to the development of science and medicine. Before the Egyptian culture, healers used witchcraft to drive out evil spirits from the body which were blamed for causing disease. The Ancient Egyptian doctors were the first physicians to study the human body scientifically. They studied the structure of the brain and knew that the pulse was in some way connected with the heart. In addition, they became masters at setting bones, caring for wounds and successfully treating many illnesses.

. The early Egyptian artists contribute to our knowledge of the medical procedures of their time. They carefully observed and recorded scenes of daily life which included the medical practices of the day. Their medical wall paintings and engravings preserve the history of surgical operations, anatomical observation and medical treatments. Both papyri and wall painting are witness to the part played by medicine and physicians in that culture.

The fame of the Egyptian medical practitioners was recognized throughout the known world at that time. Dr. Paul Ghaliongui writes:

"The prestige that surrounded the medical corps was so immense that it radiated all around Egypt and that, not only did Syrian and Persian kings resort to specialists of the Nile Valley, but that the latter shone in the eyes of the Greeks themselves with a kind of legendary glory."[4]

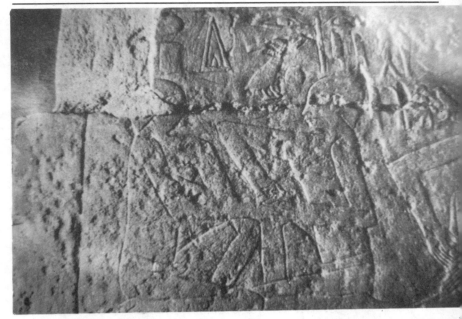

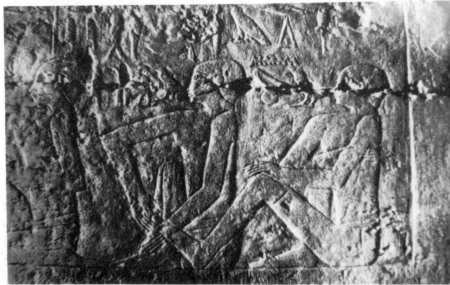

Fig. 1
Photograph of a portion of the pictograph on the wall
of the tomb of Ankhmahor.

Further evidence that the medical profession was held in great esteem is the tomb of Ankhmahor, a physician who was the most influential official, second only to the king. It is in his tomb at Saqqara that the scene depicting the practice of reflexology can be found. Egyptian physicians did not only practice medicine. Some physicians were also engineers, architects, master builders, metaphysicians, astrologers, and scribes. The knowledge a physician had, and was entitled to practice, was painted or engraved on the walls of his tomb. Ankhmahor's tomb has six wall carvings which include circumcision, child birth, pharmacology, embalming, dentistry and reflexology. These scenes were carved not only to honor the physician but also for religious purposes.

It was believed that when the spirit or soul of the physician sought to return to the body from the Afterlife it was guided by the information on the tomb walls to the correct body. Since there were many physicians, the scenes which record the activities of a person's life were, to the soul, like reading that person's biography. They aided the soul in selecting the proper body as it returned to earth.

This particular wall scene is a raised relief, without color, carved into the tomb wall. As one stands in the tomb at the opening between two chambers, the scene of circumcision, which was performed at puberty, is on the left side of the doorway and the reflexology scene is on the same wall on the right side of the passage way. To better understand the pictograph some knowledge of the Egyptian culture is helpful.

Geographically, Ancient Egypt was a long narrow country founded along the banks of the Nile. The Nile flowed north out of central Africa through the Egyptian desert to the Mediterranean Sea. Lower Egypt, to the north, was the delta region near the Mediterranean. Upper Egypt, which included the main capital of Thebes, was the area to the south towards Nubia and Central Africa. According to Egyptian Mohamed elAwany of Visions Travel and Tours, in ancient Egypt, the advanced civilization and knowledge came from the South where the darker skin was prized.

Explaining the pictograph, elAwany says, "Looking at the commercially reproduced scene, the dark ones, who have hair in the curly African style, are from Upper Egypt and they are obviously the practitioners. They have come from the south to treat those from Lower Egypt

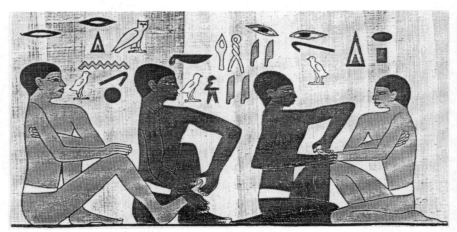

Fig. 2
Commercial reproduction of the pictograph.

who have lighter colored bodies and straight hair."

Comments elAwany, "Notice how the position of the patients is different. The patient on the left has his right hand on his right knee and his left hand under his right arm pit. The other patient is the opposite. There is a relationship between the kind of problem the patient has and where the practitioner touches. This determines the points of pressure he and the patient use. In this case, the physician is touching the toe or thumb and the patient is touching the reflex point under his arm where he feels the corresponding pain."[5]

According to the Papyrus Institute in Cairo, the hieroglyphic above the scene reads:

"Do not let it be painful," says one of the patients. "I do as you please," an attendant replies.

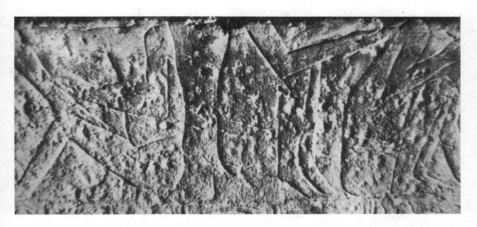

Fig. 3
Another portion of the pictograph showing
practitioners working on the lower leg and shoulder.

This pictograph is only part of the scene in the pyramid. The therapeutic application of pressure also includes the hands and the shoulders. Notes Dr. Ghaliongui, "It has been suggested they (the pictographs) represent manicure and pedicure, in spite of the fact that the hand of the practitioner, applied to the shoulder, and to the knee, rule out this possibility, and strongly suggest that they represent some form of massage or of manipulation."[6]

In order to continue tracing the spread of reflexology we must return again to Egyptian history. Ancient Egypt declined rapidly after 1,000 B.C. Finally in 332 B.C. Egypt was conquered and added to the empire of Alexander the Great. On the Nile delta, Alexander founded the city Alexandria. After Alexander died his Greek general, Ptolemy ruled Egypt. Ptolemy spread Greek culture in Egypt. Under his rule the great library of Alexandria was founded. The library had a copy of every existing papyrus scroll known. Although there is no solid evidence, it is entirely possible that the library held among its medical scrolls several on reflexology. Unfortunately nothing remains of the library at Alexandria to prove this theory. It is known, however, that the Ptolemies borrowed books from libraries in Athens and other cities and had them copied. In all likelihood some reciprocal agreement was made, and it is possible that over the centuries the practice of reflexology migrated slowly, as Dr. Riley asserts, from Egypt to Greece, Arabia and then on to Europe through the Roman Empire.

Medical knowledge in Europe remained static for centuries. During this time Islamic and Arabian doctors were responsible for preserving Greek medicine. They translated into Arabic all the Greek medical manuscripts they could obtain. One of the greatest contributions made by the Arabs was the introduction of pharmacology. In connection with this migration of medical knowledge it would appear that Dr. Riley's claim that reflexology was known in ancient Arabia is probably historically accurate.

INDIA AND CHINA

*M*as Watanabe, who is in his seventies, has for years practiced what he terms nerve therapy or Soku Shinjutsu. Soku Shinjutsu literally means, "observation of feet and treatment of foot nerves." He learned this relative of reflexology as a young student in Japan. Says Watanabe, "The history is simple. It started in India, was brought to China by Buddhist monks and then came to Japan. I studied it more than fifty years ago in a Buddhist monastery in Japan."[7]

In essence he is quite correct about the history. As happens throughout history, concepts do not appear only in one culture. The art of reflexology was not only known in Egypt but it was also known 5,000 years ago in ancient India.

The cultures of Asia have been shaped by religion, namely Hinduism and Buddhism. Hinduism, the major religion of India, is one of the oldest religions in the world. Its roots date to prehistoric times. The Hindus worship many divinities. The three most important gods are Brahma, the creator of the universe; Vishnu, its preserver; and Shiva, its destroyer. The art of India reflects the influences of Hinduism. Various temple shrines portray the divinities in sculptured images and in paintings.

In the painting titled Vishnu-padas the author Ajit Mookerjee says the feet symbolize the unity of the entire universe. He feels all the elements of the universe are represented by the signs and they also indicate the many aspects of the Ultimate One. Mookerjee explains, "As fundamentally all things are one since they are only fragments of the Supreme Unity, they are to be regarded as symbols or emblems of a higher reality."[8] This concept is not far from that held by most reflexologists that the feet (a microcosm) are a mirror of the macrocosm (the body).

Many of the Sanskrit symbols can be identified and translated by modern scholars but the true significance of them has been lost over time. Though the placement of the symbols in this and other foot print carvings and painting corresponds closely to various reflex points there is no evidence that they are connected with human anatomy. However, the placement is so exact it goes beyond coincidence. The many examples found also leaves room for doubt. Perhaps they are not meant to be exact anatomical drawings, but the aim was to show the relationship between the point location and their effects. Could it be that these images were

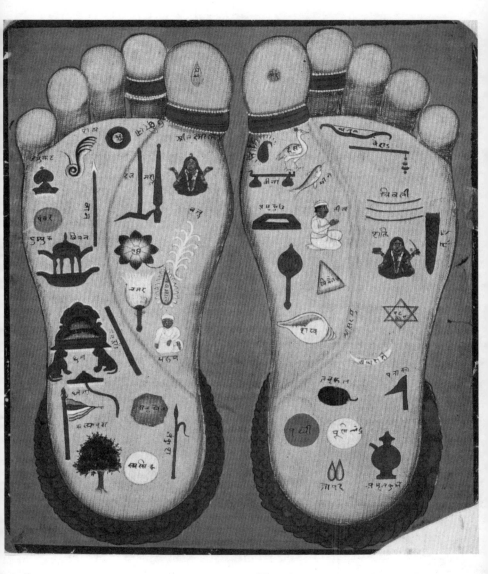

Fig. 4
India c. 18th century, The feet of Vishnu

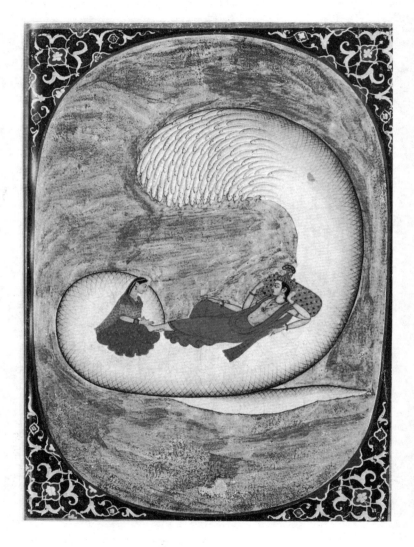

Fig. 5
India c. 1760, Lord Vishnu reclining

created not only to honor a god, but to record and impart knowledge to an illiterate society?

Buddhism

*I*n the 500's and 400's B.C. Buddha Siddhartha Guatama lived in northeastern India. Guatama through his spiritual search developed his own beliefs regarding enlightenment and preached them in his Noble Eightfold Path. He gradually attracted disciples. After his death his followers collected his traditions and developed schools and Buddhist communities composed of both monks and the laity.

At various times Buddhism has been a dominant religious, cultural and social force in India, China, Japan, Korea, Vietnam and Tibet. In each area Buddhism has combined with elements of other religions including in India with Hinduism. During the first thousand years of Indian culture from the 500's B.C. to the A.D. 500's Indian sculpture shows the influence of the Buddhist religion. By the end of the 100's A.D. Buddhism had spread to China. When we follow this migration of Buddhism one can see how reflexology could have travelled from India with the Buddhist monks to China.

Evidence may also support this theory. Several examples have been found of Buddha's footprints. In Kusinara, China there is a foot print carved into a rock and again at the Tien-tai monastery near Beijing.

According to the history traced by the Rwo Shur Health Method of Foot Reflexology (See

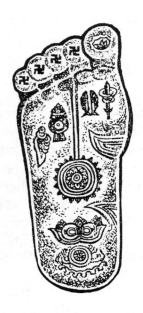

Fig. 6
Buddha's footprint
Temple at Kusinara, China

figure 9 for a flow chart of their interpretation
of the historical development of reflexology), a form
of reflexology originated in China about 4,000
years ago under Emperor Hwang as part of
Chinese acupuncture and moxibustion. The
roots of reflexology can be traced to the Chinese
medical book *Hwang Tee Internal Text* where it
is called the "Examining Foot Method". This
work is also known as "The Yellow Emperor's
Classic of Internal Medicine" or "Nei Ching" and
is attributed to Huang Ti, the Yellow Emperor
who died in 2598 B.C. The book may even date
back to 1000 B.C. because at this time author-
ship was credited to the Emperor as a way of

honoring him and is therefore not an indication of its true author or age.

As it is in the West, the history of reflexology in the Orient is often mixed with that of massage. During the Qin Dynasty (221-206 B.C.), when the Great Wall was built, Chi Po wrote four books on clinical massage. This is possibly the oldest source of massage therapy in China. However, under Emperor Shi Hunangdi most books were banned in an attempt to silence critics, to promote obedience, and to blot out knowledge of the past. At this point, according to the Rwo Shur Method the art of reflexology was nearly lost.

It was during the Han period (220-202 B.C.) that Buddhism was introduced into China. Later from 317-589 A.D., it influenced all aspects of Chinese life. By the time of the Han Dynasty, which linked China with Europe through overland trade routes, a doctor Hau To studied "Examining Foot Method" and termed it "Tao of Foot Centre" in his work *Hua Tus Mi Ji.*

The next great period in Chinese history was the Tang Dynasty (618-907 A.D.). This was an age of prosperity and great cultural accomplishment in China. The Tang capital at Chang'an (now Xian) had more than a million people. It attracted diplomats, traders, poets and scholars from throughout Asia and the Mediterranean area. Buddhism remained an enormous cultural influence. In the time of the Tang Dynasty it is recorded that "A Japanese monk, Tai Tien Chiu Shao and others studied in China. They were aware of the effectiveness of the clinical massage and introduced it to Japan."[9] Another writer in the same source indicates reflexology continued to be included within acupuncture and moxibustion.

The Mongol leader Kubali Khan established the Yuan Dynasty (1279-1368 A.D.). During the Yuan period, Fu Tai Pi Lieh wrote *Cheng Lan*

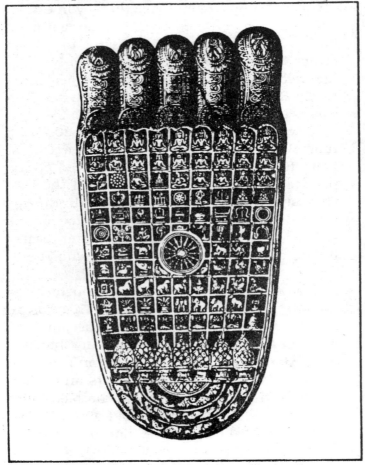

Fig. 7
Foot of Buddha

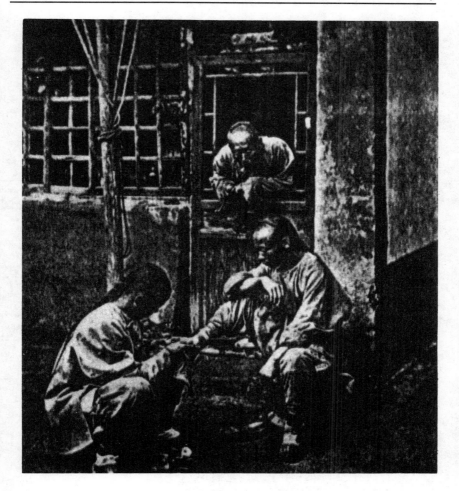

Fig. 8
Foot work in Shangai c. 1870

Chin Ching and introduced massage techniques
to Japan. At this point the Fourteen Meridian
theory, Hua Per Ren, was developed which fur-
thered the study of massage techniques.[10]

Europeans became increasingly interested
in China during the Yuan Dynasty because of

ORIGIN & DEVELOPMENT OF
RWO SHUR HEALTH METHOD

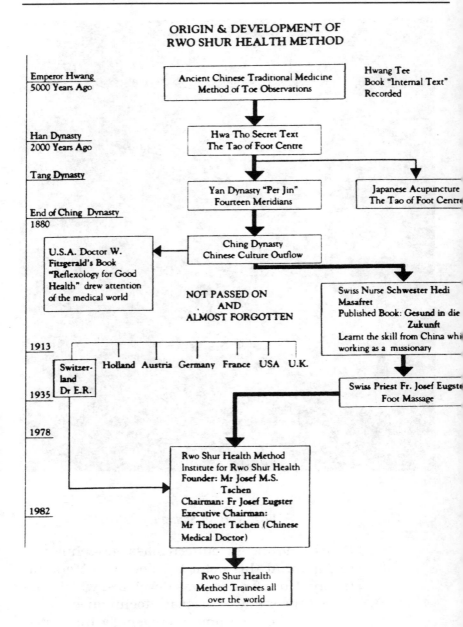

Fig. 9

the reports of travelers and traders. The most enthusiastic reports came from Marco Polo of Venice. After travelling widely in China from 1275-1292 Polo returned home with glowing reports of the highly civilized country he called Cathay. His book *A Trip to the East* gave Europeans their first information about China. *The New History of the Yuan Dynasty* states that Polo also translated the *Cheng Lan Chin Ching* in Europe. According to Master Chiao Chang Hung, "In the book there is evidence of the introduction of Chinese massage techniques to the West."[11]

Also it should be noted that Dominican and Franciscan missionaries travelled to China and were welcomed by Kubali Khan in Cambaluc (Beijing). Therefore, it is difficult to say conclusively whether reflexology came to Europe as a result of the church missionaries, Marco Polo, or both. However, it is quite evident that the two streams, one from the East and one from the West (Egypt), did converge in Europe sometime during the Dark Ages.

EUROPE

*D*uring the Middle or Dark Ages (400-1400 A.D.), very little creative or original work was conceived. The feudal system controlled secular life, and education was under the dominance of the church. Medicine made little progress and was practiced mainly in the learning centers of the monasteries. The monks grew herbs for use as medicine. They did collect and study the work of Greek and Roman doctors. However, as scholars, they were more interested in theology than the study of nature and medicine.

Finally, in the second half of the 14th century there was an increase in the number of scholars who were not clerics. This occurred with the invention of the Gutenberg printing press which allowed the works of Galen—200-130 B.C., a Greek physician who had studied in Alexandria—and others to be read more widely outside religious circles. During the Renaissance, artist Leonardo da Vinci (1452-1519) also contributed to medicine. He was the first to draw accurate pictures of the human anatomy from cadavers.

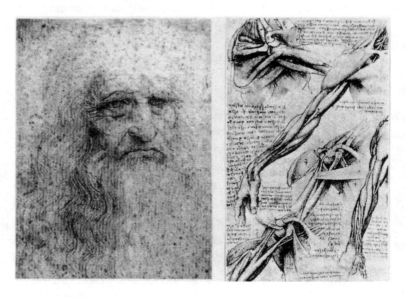

Fig. 10
Self portait of Leonardo da Vinci and sketches of the muscles in the shoulder and arm from his notebook.

The beginning of the modern period of science starts with Descartes. Rene Descartes (1596-1650), French philosopher, mathematician and scientist was a pioneer in separating the world into two kinds of substances—matter and spirit. He felt man's mind had to be excluded from the physical body or the mechanical sphere. Descartes suggested that the body could be studied by the use of quantitative techniques, but the mind only through the process of meditation. The scientific-material thought process had been born. An eventual consequence of his theories was a less holistic approach to the treatment of disease. Of course, Descartes, like all original thinkers in any age, was opposed by the popular beliefs of the day, but it is this stream of thought—the separation of man into a physical body and a mind—that science eventually followed. This allowed for a rapid advancement in the field of medicine.

Until recently, it was thought that the concept of reflexology was largely unknown by Western Civilization. In Europe, a form of reflexology called zone therapy was known and practiced. Zone therapy relieves pain and stress with the application of pressure to zones of the body. The pressure causes a reflex action to occur in another part of the same zone. According to Harry Bond Bressler in his book *Zone Therapy*:

"Pressure therapy was well known in the middle countries of Europe and was practiced by the working classes of those countries as well as by those who catered to the diseases of

Royalty and the upper classes. Dr. Adamus and Dr. A'tatis wrote a book on the subject of zone therapy which was published in 1582. In Leipsig Dr. Ball wrote another book on the same subject, and it was published soon after the other book."[12]

The scientific stream of medicine was also aided by the Industrial Revolution of the 1750's. This was a time of invention. The invention of diagnostic tools, like the microscope, took precedence over theory. Three hundred years after Descartes' separation of man into body and mind, his ideas were further developed by Charles Darwin (1809-1882) into the theory of evolution. Darwin published his idea on natural selection through competition, or survival of the fittest, in 1858. With its strong emphasis on the physical, Darwin's theory revolutionized biological science and greatly affected religious thought. Medical science made several breakthroughs. A handful of new sciences had their beginning in the 1800's, while older disciplines separated into smaller areas of concentration. Physiology branched off of biology, and later, psychology branched off physiology. With the advent of Darwinism, research with animals accelerated. Evolutionary thinking modified psychological perspectives regarding sensation-perception and association.

A few years before Darwin, Johann August Unzer (1747-1807), a German physiologist was the first to use the word "reflex" with reference to motor reactions in his work published in 1771. This was followed in 1833 with the introduction of the concept and the term "reflex action" by Marshall Hall (1790-1857), an English physiologist. Hall also demonstrated the difference between unconscious reflexes and volitional acts in a study on the reflex function of the medulla oblongata and the spinal cord.

In those early years, and even today, many areas of science overlap with scientists in several fields studying the same problem from different points of view. Often it is difficult to make clear-cut definitions as to where one science begins and another ends. For example, psychology is concerned with the behavior of man and animals. Some psychologists may work with medical scientists to study the causes of mental nervous diseases, while others are concerned with the relationship between behavior and the function of the nervous system, including the various organs of the body. At the same time neurologists study how the nervous system works and reacts to stimuli. In yet another way, philosophers turn their focus on various aspects of human experience. The philosopher's concern with how man can adjust to his changing world, can overlap with the field of psychology.

The scientific study of why human beings and animals behave as they do began in the mid-1800's. Research indicates that the scientific basis of reflexology has its roots in early neurological studies conducted in the 1890's by Sir Henry Head of London. Head worked with Nobel prize winner, Sir Charles Sherrington. According to Kevin and Barbara Kunz, "during this time (the 1890's) whole schools of thought, research efforts and published articles were directed toward the reflex of man's reaction to his environment."[13] These schools were to include some of the outstanding scientists of the time and provoke many arguments among them.

CHAPTER 2

MODERN EUROPEAN HISTORY
1850 - 1962

THE BRITISH

$\mathcal{N}$eurology is a recent field of medicine dealing widely with the organization and functioning of the brain and nervous system. Although research was going on in this area it was not until the late 1880's that it became a field of its own. The Neurological Society of London was founded with the object of promoting the advance of neurology and to facilitate communication among those who were interested in the field whether from a psychological, physiological, anatomical or pathological point of view. Corresponding members hailed from all over Europe, with the United States having one representative. Three of the founding members, John Huglings Jackson, Sir Henry Head and Sir Charles Sherrington put forth theories that would dominate the field for the next fifty years.

Each member received a quarterly copy of *Brain, A Journal of Neurology*. Periodically articles regarding the most up-to-date research on reflex action were published. In 1878 *Brain* published an article by Dr. T. Lauter Brunton titled: *"Reflex Action As A Cause of Disease and Means of Cure"*. Brunton discussed the beneficial use of inducing a blister on the skin for the healing of internal problems, citing: "the blister acts reflexly upon the organ itself." To illustrate his point he says, "A blister to the heel will sometimes afford relief, while applied in the neighbourhood of the nerve itself has little or no effect."[1]

In 1893 M.J. Babinski, a French physician, wrote the paper *"A Phenomenon Of The Toes and Its Symptomatological Value"*. In the paper he was the first to prove how dorsiflexion of the big toe and fanning of the other toes occurred when the sole of the foot is scraped. Later, in 1896, he reported on additional findings in a paper he wrote titled: *"Plantar Cutaneous Reflexes in Certain Organic Conditions of the Central Nervous System"*.[2]

John Hughlings Jackson (1835-1911), under the influence of Darwin's theory of evolution, theorized that the nervous system was composed of different levels organized in such a way that the level above restrained and regulated the activities of the level below it. Expanding on this theory, Sir Henry Head wrote a paper

BRAIN.

PARTS I. & II., 1893.

Original Articles.

ON DISTURBANCES OF SENSATION WITH ESPECIAL REFERENCE TO THE PAIN OF VISCERAL DISEASE.[1]

BY HENRY HEAD, M.A., M.D.

University College Hospital.

INTRODUCTORY.

SEVERAL years ago I was led to examine the positions occupied by pain in disorders of the stomach and I soon came to the conclusion that the usual description was incomplete in several respects. For firstly the positions over which the patient experienced pain in gastric disturbances were more numerous than was usually supposed, and secondly the pain was in many cases associated with definite cutaneous tenderness. Moreover the cutaneous tenderness was in many cases not confined to small spots or areas, but occupied whole tracts of skin with definite borders. I was thus led to investigate the pain and accompanying tenderness consequent on disturbances of other organs, and I found that these sensory disturbances also followed definite lines.

After Ross's most suggestive papers it seemed exceedingly probable that these areas bore some definite relation to nerve distribution, and I then began to investigate the distribution of herpes zoster in the hope that a skin lesion which was notoriously of nervous origin might throw some light ' on the meaning and significance of the tender areas in visceral

[1] Read as a Thesis before the University of Cambridge, June, 1892, and before the Neurological Society of London, November 10th, 1892.

VOL. XVI.   1

Fig. 11

for *Brain* in 1893 titled, *"On Disturbances of Sensation With Especial Reference to the Pain of Visceral Disease"*. With the help of patients who had traumatic lesions of the spinal cord Head was able to chart areas according to the spinal segment to which it belonged. He found the whole body and limbs could be marked into areas which correspond to the distribution of the pain given off from one segment of the spinal cord. After years of clinical research Head established what became known as "Head's zones" or "zones of hyperalgesia". Head charted areas of skin sensitiveness associated with diseases of the internal organs. He writes, "I was enabled to map out the areas supplied by the various segments of the cord on the surface of the body." Later in the same work he states, "These areas do not overlap one another, and it is a peculiar characteristic of these areas of painful sensation that wherever they are situated on the surface of the body, whether they be marked out by hyperalgesia or analgesia, their limits never materially alter or overlap."[3]

In his experimental research Head went so far as to use himself as a subject. He and fellow physician, W.H.R. Rivers, cut a nerve in Head's left forearm and reported on the results of their study in *Brain* under the title of *"The Afferent Nervous System from a New Aspect."*[4] Head's and River's study of the loss and restoration of sensation brought about a re-classification of the sensory pathways. In conjunction with this study Head decided the body organized the sensibility to pain on three different levels— "deep" sensibility came as a response to pressure and movement; "protopathic" sensibility was somewhat primitive and was a vague response to extremes of heat, cold and pain; and "epicritic" or normal sensibility was accurate and discriminating for all forms of skin stimulation.[5]

Head conclusively proved the neurological relationship that exists between the skin and internal organs. He writes in *Aphasia and Kindred Disorders*, "The bladder can be excited to action by stimulating the sole of the foot, and movements of the toes can be evoked by filling the bladder with fluid."[6] Head's work on the

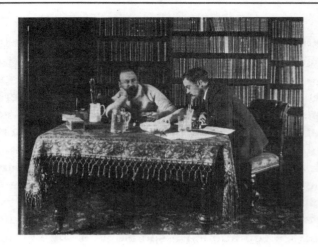

Fig. 12
Sir Henry Head (r.) and W.H.R. Rivers (l.)

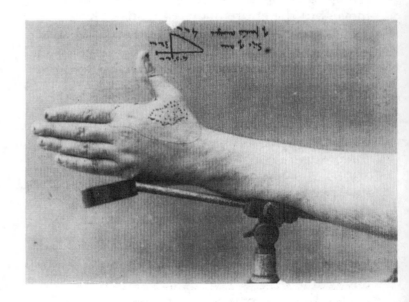

Fig. 13
Head's illustration from his report on the restoration
of sensation

sensory functions of the skin was taught in medical schools for years.

Sir Charles Sherrington (1861-1952) did for reflex action what Head had done for the sensation of pain. At the same time Head was running his experiments, his friend Sherrington was investigating and proving that stimuli are produced within the organism by movement in its own tissue, especially from a reflex aspect. He termed this the proproceptive system. Unlike the Russians, Sherrington did not see conditioned response as a simple arc. Instead he proved that the whole nervous system adjusts to a stimulus. For instance, when a step is taken, not only does the foot and leg move, but the entire body responds to keep the body upright. Sherrington insisted that the essential function of the nervous system was the coordination of activities of the various parts of the organism.

Sherrington's work on the reflex action of the nervous system greatly influenced modern physiology. He published his classic work *The Integrative Action of the Nervous System* in 1906. This book explains how the nerves coordinate and dominate body functions. He showed the process by which the brain, spinal cord and numerous reflex pathways control the activities of the body. Through this reflex action the entire body adjusts to a stimulus or the environment.

In 1932, Sherrington's work earned him the Nobel Prize. He shared the Nobel Prize with Edgar Adrian for their work on the physiology of the nervous system. Adrian also made a

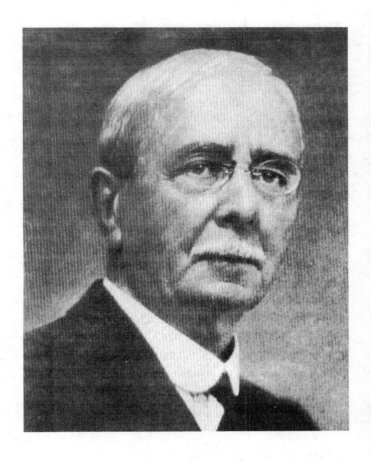

Fig. 14
Nobel Prize winner, Sir Charles Sherrington

discovery that all reflexologists should be aware
of. Not long after World War I, he showed that
the electrical intensity of the nerve impulse de-
pended on the size of the nerve rather than upon
the strength of the stimulus.

English scientists continued to explore neurology. Thirty-one years after Sherrington and Adrian another pair of British researchers, Hodgkin and Huxley, would be awarded the Nobel Prize for their neurological work. In 1963 the two were awarded the Nobel Prize for their description of the behavior and transmission of nerve impulses.

THE GERMANS

Reflexzonenmassage

*G*erman physicians specializing in the treatment of disease by massage have left behind many works on the subject. In the late 1890's and early 1900's massage techniques were developed in Germany that became known as "reflex massage." This was the first time that the benefits of massage techniques were credited to reflex actions.

According to Herman Kamenetz, Dr. Alfons Cornelius "was probably the first to apply massage to "reflex zones" even though he was apparently unfamiliar with the work of Henry Head."[7] The story goes that in 1893 Cornelius suffered from an infection. In the course of his convalescence he received a daily massage. At the spa he noticed how effective the massages of one particular medical officer were. This man worked longer on areas that he found painful. This concept inspired Cornelius. After examining himself Cornelius instructed his masseur to work only on the painful areas. His pain quickly disappeared and in four weeks he completely recovered. This led him to pursue the use of pressure in his own medical practice.

Cornelius published his manuscript, *Druck-punkte*, or *Pressure Points, Their Origin and Significance* in 1902. "The name pressure point is not quite accurate for these points,"[8] writes the doctor. The localized areas of sensitivity, Cornelius discovered, not only responded to pressure but the application of pressure also incited other changes to occur in the body. He observed pressure to certain spots triggered muscle contraction, changes in blood pressure, variation in warmth and moisture in the body as well as directly affecting the "psychic processes" or mental state of the patient. He also notes, "These (points) are already long since known in medicine."[9] Cornelius also established that the pressure points worked within the nerve pathways, following the anatomy of the body. He did find, however, there were some exceptions to this purely anatomical concept. Dr. Cornelius maintained the consequences of pressure was "a purely mechanical hindering of the sensitive neurons, the neurons of the sympathetic nerve system."[10] He likened the results that could be achieved to the laws of acoustics. "One tone can in turn call forth another tone with the similar number of oscillations. Then I have come to the conclusion that analogue to the nerve agitation that race through the body, in a similar way to the sensitive points of the nerves, such a reaction can be released. With the help of such a hypothesis it is possible for me to explain the truly remarkably high number of reactions of far distant pressure points working all the way from the top of the skull to the bottom of the foot."[11]

Cornelius, like Henry Head, charted out different classifications of pain according to intensity; and the amount of pressure applied to stimulate the healing process. He found pressure points on the surface of the body in the skin, and deeper in the musculature. In addition, he discovered two other types of painful sensations. The first was a radiating pain, which spread out from the pressure point and was not bound to anatomical law. This pain sometimes jumped over the parts of the body. "If at one pressure point it is possible, whether it lies near or far away to bring forth a pain at quite a distant part of the body, then at all circumstances this particular place is in itself a further pressure point."[12] The last, and rarest type of pain, he describes is a point which radiates in a starry form and does not indicate any further pressure points. One other interesting occurrence he noted was that all conditions show themselves as sensitive pressure points and "introduce the picture of illness long before it is to be recognized as an expression of a neurological problem."[13]

Cornelius found that not all parts of the body respond at the same rate. He writes, "the pressure points in the back of the head, then on the feet, and in the inter rib spaces, present the greatest continuity and difficulties. The duration they require to come to total lack of sensitivity varies from eight days to five months."[14]

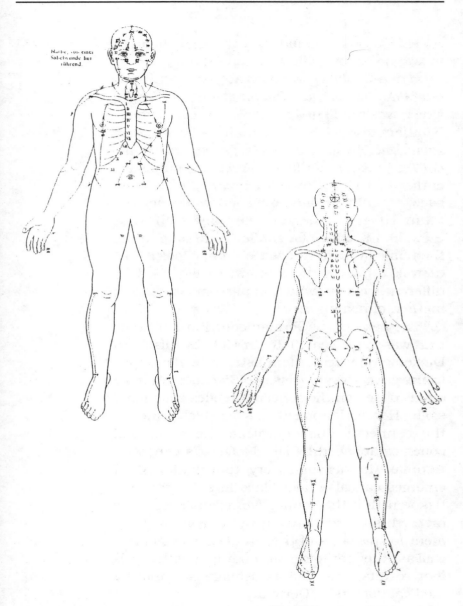

Fig. 15
Clinical chart showing pressure points by Dr. Alfons Cornelius, 1902

Dr. Cornelius found support for his theories in two books by other German authors. *Treatment and Healing of Nervous Suffering and Nervous Pain by Hand Manipulation*, by Naegeli which was published in 1899. A second source he refers to is Algien Benedikts' book, *On Neuralgia and Neurologic Effects, Questions of Clinical Treatment and Clinical Problems*, published earlier in 1892. Cornelius taught "nerve massage" techniques only to his fellow physicians.

In 1911, another German physician, Barczewski, introduced a similar technique under the name of "Reflexmassage" in his book. Barczewski's use of the term was then used by different systems which applied pressure as a method of healing.[15]

The next major German contribution to the field was made years later in 1929 by Elisabeth Dicke, a physical therapist. She developed Connective Tissue Massage *(Bindegewebsmassage)*, based on the concept of reflex zone massage. Her work applied massage techniques to the connective tissue within the segmental zones established by Head. Dicke's contribution lies in her discovery that pathological changes can also take place in subcutaneous tissue within the connective tissue layer. Her method is currently used not only as a treatment for diseases of the circulatory system as well as other pathological conditions with excellent results, but also as a diagnostic tool by medical doctors in Germany.

In 1955 W. Kohlrausch in his book *Reflexzonenmassage in Muskulatur und Bindegewebe* discussed changes to the skin associated with disturbances of the organs as well as the therapeutic effect which massage and exercise have on the condition of diseased organs. He felt that disturbances of the organs follow vascular channels which are associated with the reflexes of the arteries. The theory of these channels would account for the many structual and functional changes which cannot be explained as a result of reflex action within the segmental nervous system. Kolhrausch believes that the disappearance of symptoms when Compression Massage Therapy is applied to the back, even though the back segments treated do not correspond to the dermatome area, supports his conclusion.[16]

Finally, Hanne Marquardt, after training in the United States with Eunice Ingham in 1970, took German reflex zone therapy one step further with pressure being applied only to the feet. Her book *Reflex Zone Therapy of the Feet* was first published in 1974. Marquardt like Cornelius restricts her teaching to medical personnel. Regarding Marquardt's work, Dr. Erich Rauch states, "Mrs. Marquardt proved the value of treatment of the feet for such a wide range of ailments that it has since become a quite indispensable form of treatment amongst us. These include: disorders of the musculo-skeletal system and the spine; functional disorders of the respiratory and genito-urinary systems; developmental disorders of childhood, and several others. Many rare conditions are amenable to treatment with this method provided that their reflex signature has been visibly and palpably engraved on the relevant foot zone."[17]

THE SOVIETS

Reflextoinaya Therapiya

𝒫sychology is concerned with the behavior of the whole organism while physiology, the closest other science, has to do with the functioning of the parts of the body. Often the two disciplines intertwine, with scientists making contributions in both fields. Such was the case with the Russians.

The Russian work with reflexes began more from a psychological point of view. The founder of Russian physiology was Ivan Sechenov. Sechenov was professor of physiology at St. Petersburg and later in Moscow. He discovered the cerebral inhibition of spinal reflexes. Around 1870 Sechenov published the paper, *"Who Must Investigate the Problems of Psychology and How?"* The psychologists under the leadership of Vladimir Bekhterev picked up the challenge and studied it through the reflexes.

During the same time Ivan Pavlov (1849-1936) read Sechenov's work and acknowledged that his book *Reflexes of the Brain* was the most important theoretical inspiration for his own work on conditioning. Pavlov took Sechenov's theoretical outline and submitted it to methodical experimental study. Through this, Pavlov developed the theory of conditioned reflexes, namely that there is a simple and direct relationship between a stimulus and a response.

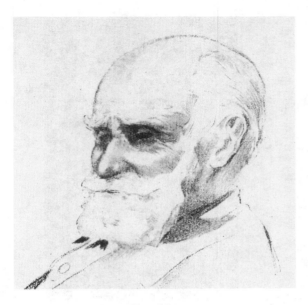

Fig. 16
Dr. Ivan Pavlov

Pavlov found practically any stimulus can act
as a conditioning stimulus to produce a conditioned response. In 1904 he was awarded the
Nobel Prize for his discovery of the secretory
nerves of the pancreas.

In the early years of his work public arguments existed between Pavlov and his contem-
porary Bekhterev. Bekhterev, who had greater
influence at the time, was more a psychiatrist
than a physiologist and carried into psychology
the conception of the objective method of studying the complex functions of the brain which
Pavlov had introduced in physiology. Bekhterev actually originated the term "reflexology".[18] In 1907 he published a series of

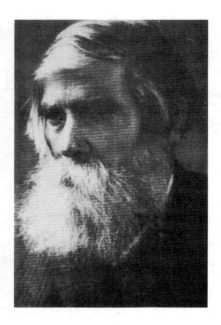

Fig. 17
Dr. Vladimir Bekhterev

lectures under the title, *Objective Psychology*. This work was translated into German and French in 1913 and finally into English in 1932 under his revised title of *General Principles of Human Reflexology*. Bekhterev's opening sentence defines reflexology far differently than modern day reflexologists would. He writes:

"Reflexology, which is a new doctrine, is the science of human personality studied from the strictly objective, bio-social standpoint. It embraces a special sphere of knowledge to which human thought has not yet become accustomed, and consists in investigating, from the strictly objective standpoint, not only the more elementary, but also all the higher, functions of the human being, which in everyday language are called the manifestations of feeling, knowing, and willing, or, speaking generally, the phenomena of psychic activity—the 'spiritual sphere.' In this way it confines itself to the external peculiarities of the activity of man: his facial expressions, his gestures, voice, and speech as a coherent integration of signs, in correlation with the exciting external influences—physical, biological, and, above all, social—but also with the internal, regardless of whether either of these two types of influence is referable to the present or the past."[19]

In his papers he argued for the application of the objective approach to the problems of psychology. This objective approach he felt was sufficient enough to account for man's behavior.

Bekhterev founded Leningrad's Brain Institute. Over the years the Institute appears to have changed it's reflexology research emphasis from a psychological viewpoint to a physical one. His granddaughter Natalia, as director of the Institute in 1978, reports, "researchers of the Brain Institute have pinpointed and explored two thousand zones of the brain, each serving a different purpose. This was accomplished parallel with the Institute's hospital work of diagnosing and treating patients."[20]

Since the Revolution of 1917, Soviet scientific endeavors have remained largely unknown to the West, because most Westerners do not read Russian and the Soviets choose not to associate and exchange ideas freely with the

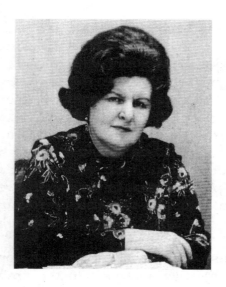

Fig. 18
Dr. Natalia Bekhterev

West. Perhaps with the fall of communism this situation will change.

The Soviets, however, did pursue the study of reflexology both from the physiological and psychological point of view. This is evidenced by the large number of articles published by them and other Soviet block countries on the subject—more than one hundred in the last twenty years. They have scientifically tested the effect of reflex therapy on patients with a variety of problems.

One center for such studies is the Leningrad Sanitary-Hygiene Medical Institute founded by a pupil of Pavlov's, Nikolai Yakovevich Ketcher. In Volume 60 of the Institute's publication, all the articles are related to reflex therapy being applied to pathological problems of the digestive organs or to those of the cardiovascular system. Reports the editor, G.N. Udintsev, "The article entitled *'Relationship between muscle tone and arterial pressure'* was written by A.I. Makarova, instructor in the department of physical training and medical grading, and consultant in our clinic on the application of physical exercise to patients with various diseases, including hypertension. Without summarizing the observations and the relevant conditions, we may merely state that Makarova recognizes the presence of reflex relationship between the cardiovacular system and the skeletal musculature, that stimulation of the interoceptors affects muscle tone and stimulation of the proprioceptors has consistent effects on the circulatory system..."[21]

Published Soviet articles indicate the Russians have used reflexology in conjunction with bronchial asthma, influenza, obstetrics, tintinnitus (ringing in the ear), cerebral palsy and low back pain. In the USSR reflexology has been found to be an effective complement to traditional medicine.

As much as the European have contributed to reflex research it was in the United States that the techniques of reflex therapy were eventually formulated into what is commonly termed reflexology. The publishing of various American authors in foreign languages has spread the American approach world-wide.

CHAPTER 3

THE AMERICANS AND REFLEXOLOGY

"*T*he practice of massaging the reflex zones of the feet comes from ancient folk medicine. It is known to have been employed by Red Indian tribes and was probably passed down to us by the Incas, who greatly refined the old Indian techniques," writes Franz Wagner in his book *Reflex Zone Massage.* Wagner even goes so far as to claim that Dr. William Fitzgerald, who is credited with being the father of modern reflexology, first came across zone therapy as practiced by the "Red Indians". Unfortunately Wagner does not cite any sources for these statements.[1]

The Inca empire began to expand about 1438 and was conquered by Spanish forces one hundred years later. The Incas did not develop a writing system so there are no sources about them prior to the Spanish conquest. However, the Incas probably did have some kind of foot work. The Indians of North America certainly did. Pressure applied to the feet as a source of healing was used by several different Indian tribes.

Jenny Wallace, a full-blooded Cherokee Indian, from the Blue Ridge Mountains of North Carolina says that in Bear Clan—the clan of her father—feet are important. "Your feet walk upon the earth and through this your spirit is connected to the universe. Our feet are our contact with the earth and the energies that flow through it," Wallace says.

Cherokee tradition is hundreds of years old. Before the Pilgrims landed at Plymouth Rock the Cherokee nation lived as ranchers and farmers in the fertile land where the state of North Carolina is today. The Cherokees befriended the Europeans and adopted many of their ways. They were one of the most prosperous and progressive tribes in the country. During the Revolutionary War a unit composed of Cherokees fought for the British. After the war they continued farming with aid from their black slaves. However, after gold was discovered on their lands in Northern Georgia, the U.S. Government relocated the Cherokees to Oklahoma as part of its expansion policy between 1838-40. During the forced march, known to the Cherokees as the Trail of Tears, many of the estimated 16,000 who began the march died. A small band of about 1,000 refused to leave North Carolina and fled to the back hills of the Alleghanies, including the Blue Ridge Mountains. Many live there today—far off any road, without electricity or telephones, as they keep their culture intact.

Jenny Wallace grew up in such an atmosphere. She is a "moonmaiden" not a shaman. A moon maiden, she explained, is a little girl who exhibits natural intuitive healing talents and is chosen by the tribe to develop this talent further. In contrast, a shaman is one taught to heal as an adult. "All tribes are different, even within the Cherokee nation," reports Wallace. "In my tribe working on the feet is a very important healing art and is a part of sacred ceremony that you don't have to be ill to take part in. Though not living with my tribe today I still make my living working on people. First I will bathe the feet and then push any negative energy out of the body through the feet. Sometimes I work with the thumb bent and other times with it straight. A mental connection exists between the client and me. In my culture, there is no set routine so I work according to the needs of the body I am working on. I sometimes use oils on the feet—originally scented bear grease was used—and other times I don't use anything. Perhaps I will use a sage or dandelion soak and clay packs. It really all depends on the needs of my client," concluded Wallace.[2]

Jim Rolls, a ninth generation Cherokee to do reflexology learned from his great-grandfather, "Coon Dog" Henderson. Rolls' great-great-grandmother died on the Trail of Tears near Hopkinsville, Kentucky. The family settled nearby. Jim lives and practices reflexology across the border in Evansville, Indiana. "The practice of reflexology has been passed on through an apprenticeship in our family since the 1690's," Jim says. "My technique is different than what is generally taught because I apply firm straight strokes using the side of the thumb and oil, instead of the thumb walking technique employed by most reflexologists today," he continued. Jim further explains, "Traditional Indian medicine is aimed at restoring the patient to a balance with nature. I find out what is wrong in the body by working on the feet. When an area is painful on the foot I go to the corresponding part of the body and massage that area too."

The Cherokees were the only Indian nation with a written language. Chief Sequoya introduced a system of writing, using 86 symbols, in 1821 which many Cherokees learned to read and write. So many in fact that the Cherokee nation had its own newspaper. However, there is no known written record of foot work or charts among the Cherokees or any other American Indians.

On the West Coast, in at least one tribe foot work was unknown. Anna Leest, of native Hawaiian and American Indian descent, from Crescent City, California, reports her tribe, the Yuroks, did no foot work. "Hawaiians rubbed feet—they didn't know why, they just did it. I found rubbing my son's feet as a youngster helped him sleep better. I didn't actually learn reflexology until years later after I found out my brother-in-law was practicing zone therapy.

This was followed by an apprenticeship for two years with Alice Brinkley in Cave Junction, Oregon. Brinkley introduced me to the Ingham system and I studied with them. Today I combine reflexology with my intuitive feelings. My clients get different treatments based on what their bodies need," shared Leest.

Throughout America there is a strong tradition of foot work amongst Indian tribes, but whether it was passed down by Incas remains to be seen. Regardless of the origin, the work of Rolls, Wallace and Leest lends support to the theory that reflexology is an archetypal form of therapy. Also, whether Fitzgerald first came across zone therapy as practiced by the Indians remains unproven and doubtful. It seems more probable that his first contact with the theory was in Europe.

Formally, the development and practice of reflexology in the United States is a result of studies conducted by Dr. William Fitzgerald (1872-1942) in the early part of this century with zone therapy. Dr. Fitzgerald received his medical degree from the University of Vermont in 1895. He practiced in Boston City Hospital for two and a half years before going to London. He then spent two years at Central London Nose and Throat Hospital prior to taking a position in Vienna as assistant to professors Politzer and Chiari. Fitzgerald worked under highly respected doctors. Dr. Adam Politzer (1835-1920) of the University of Vienna was a well known author of many medical books and made clinical contributions to the diagnosis and treatment of diseases of the ear. Dr. Otto

Chiari, again an established authority, wrote several books on diseases and surgery for the larynx and trachea.

Fitzgerald never published where he became acquainted with the theory of zone therapy, nor does he give any credit to original sources of work preceding his. Fitzgerald also makes no reference to any Oriental influence. As cited previously, zone therapy was known in Europe in the 1500's so Fitzgerald cannot be "the discoverer of zone therapy" as Dr. Bowers claims,[3] perhaps the term "re-discoverer" would be more appropriate. According to Harry Bond Bressler in *Zone Therapy*, Fitzgerald became acquainted with the art of pressure therapy in Vienna.[4] This is entirely possible. Fitzgerald must have spoken and read German. The same year Fitzgerald was in Vienna, Cornelius, published his manuscript *Pressure Points, Their Origin and Significance*. Later, in 1909 and 1933 this work was updated and republished under the titles *Die Nervenpunktlehre (The Doctrine of Nerve Points)* and *Die Nervenpunkte (Nerve Points)*. Academic circles tend to be small, therefore, Fitzgerald could have easily heard about or read the 1902 treatise which was published at the same time he was in that city.

Another influence could have been the work of Dr. d'Arsonval. In *Zone Therapy Is Scientific* by W.D. Chesney, M.D. states, "In Germany, that great doctor, d'Arsonval was using Physio-Therapy and getting relief following the use of reflex knowledge which, in effect was what was later termed Zone Therapy by Drs. Fitzgerald and Bowers."[5] Arsende d'Arsonval was actually a French physician who published in 1914 his paper, *The Future of Medicine*, in which he states that future medical therapies will involve the use of heat, light and electricity, not drugs.

Upon his return to the U.S. Fitzgerald became head of the Nose and Throat Department of St. Francis Hospital in Hartford, Connecticut. Apparently around 1909 Fitzgerald "discovered" zone therapy. Almost ten years later in his book he writes how he stumbled upon the concept of zone therapy:

"Six years ago I accidentally discovered that pressure with a cotton-tipped probe on the muco-cutaneus margin (where the skin joins the mucus membrane) of the nose gave an anesthetic result as though a cocaine solution had been applied.

"I further found that there were many spots in the nose, mouth, throat, and on both surfaces of the tongue which, when pressed firmly, deadened definite areas of sensation. Also, that pressures exerted over any bony eminence, on the hands, feet, or over the joints, produced the same characteristic results in pain relief. I found also that when pain was relieved, the condition that produced the pain was most generally relieved. This led to my 'mapping out' these various areas and their associated connections, and also to noting the conditions influenced through them. This science I have named zone therapy."[6]

Fitzgerald began research into the use of zone therapy and used it on his patients. He verified that pressure on various parts of the body, primarily the hands, fingers, mouth and feet, could be used to bring about a numbing effect on another area. This resulted in the need for little or no anesthetic during surgery or treatment.

According to Edwin Bowers, M.D., Fitzgerald did not start out his research with any hypothesis, but simply dealt with the results that occurred with his use of pressure. Nor did he present any theories or explanation to his medical colleagues. Instead, he demonstrated clinical facts and expected those facts to convince his peers as to the effectiveness of zone therapy.[7] It is interesting to note that the reflex zones of the feet, so crucial to modern reflexology therapy, were not singled out for any special attention by Fitzgerald.

Through the knowledge he gained in Europe, and his own research, Fitzgerald theorized the body can be divided into ten longitudinal lines or zones. Fitzgerald and Head were not the only researchers to divide the body into zones. Head's zones, were further refined into dermatomes. During the same time, on the opposite side of the world in Japan, Psychologist Dr. Kurakichi Hirata in 1913 divided the body into horizontal zones.[8] His system is one of seven regions of the body further divided with twelve zones in each region. The Chinese had, in Acupuncture, divided the body into longitudinal meridians by approximately 2,500 B.C. Today, Western Chiropractic medicine also divides the spine into segments with spinal segments corresponding to the major organs and areas of the body. Apparently these discoveries were made independently in different parts of

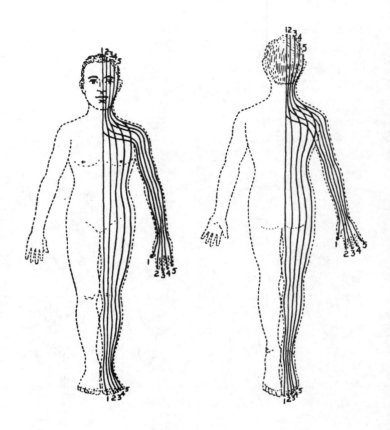

Fig. 19
Fitzgerald Zones, 1917

the world. There are no indications linking Eastern and Western zone systems although between the different Eastern systems or between the various Western systems links can be made.

Like Head, Fitzgerald found that stimulation of the skin caused a reflex action to occur. By working anywhere in a zone, everything in the zone was affected.

55

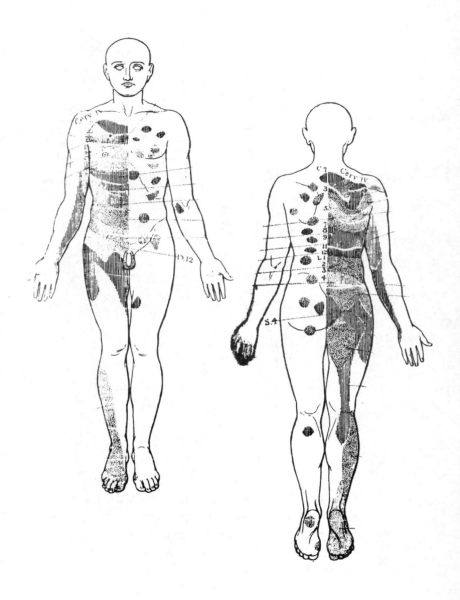

Fig. 20
Head Zones, 1893

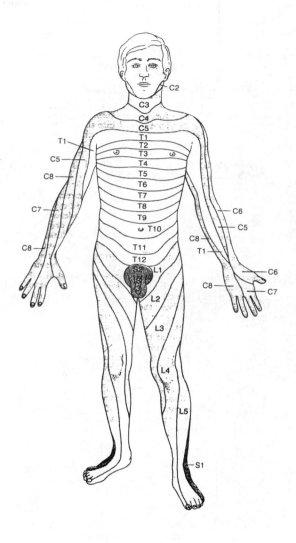

Fig. 21
Dermatomes

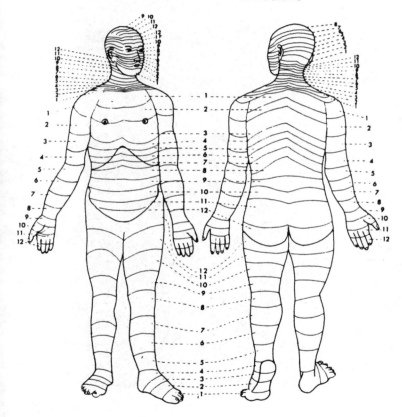

The Hirata Zones

1 TRACHEA-BRONCHI
2 LUNGS
3 HEART
4 LIVER
5 GALL BLADDER
6 SPLEEN-PANCREAS
7 STOMACH
8 KIDNEYS
9 LARGE INTESTINES
10 SMALL INTESTINES
11 URINARY BLADDER
12 GENITAL ORGANS

Fig. 22
Hirata Zones, 1913
as interpreted by Dr. Ralph Alan Dale

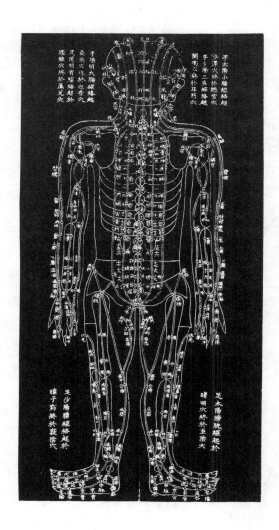

Fig. 23
Acupuncture meridians, 2,500 B.C.

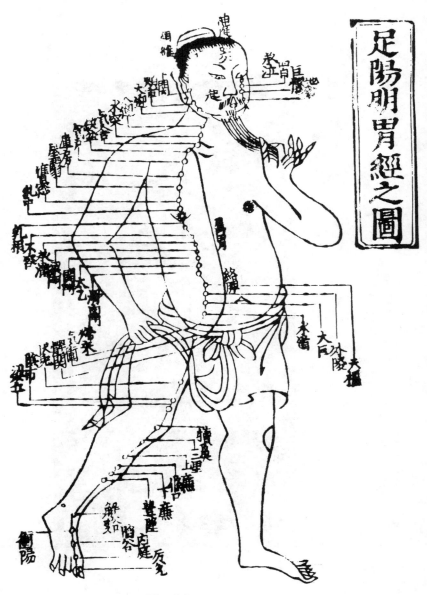

Fig. 24
Chinese acupuncture chart showing the points on the
stomach meridian

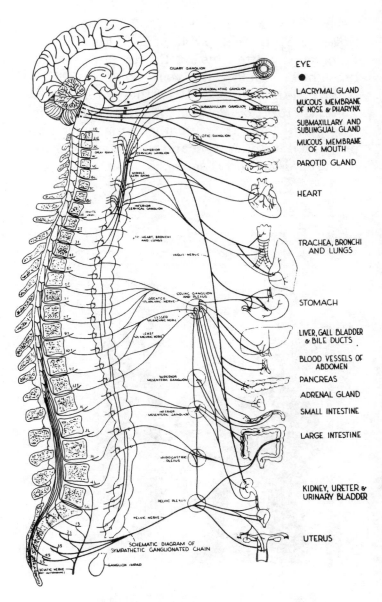

Fig. 25
Autonomic nerve control of organs and glands

In 1915 the article "To Stop That Toothache, Squeeze Your Toe" published in *Everybody's Magazine*[9] written by Dr. Edwin Bowers, first brought Dr. Fitzgerald's work on zone therapy before the public. In 1917 they co-authored *Zone Therapy or Relieving Pain in the Home*. Two years later they enlarged this book and published it under a second title, *Zone Therapy or Curing Pain and Disease*.

TO STOP THAT TOOTH-ACHE, SQUEEZE YOUR TOE!

By EDWIN F BOWERS M D

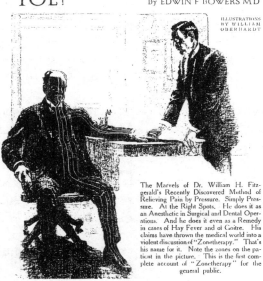

ILLUSTRATIONS
BY WILLIAM
OBERHARDT

The Marvels of Dr. William H. Fitzgerald's Recently Discovered Method of Relieving Pain by Pressure. Simply Pressure. At the Right Spots. He does it as an Anesthetic in Surgical and Dental Operations. And he does it even as a Remedy in cases of Hay Fever and of Goitre. His claims have thrown the medical world into a violent discussion of "Zonetherapy." That's his name for it. Note the zones on the patient in the picture. This is the first complete account of "Zonetherapy" for the general public.

WE GRIND and grit our teeth during paroxysms of pain. When we bump our shins against a rocking-chair that has taken point of vantage directly in our path, immediately we clasp the offended shin.

In the days before the blessed era of nitrous-oxid and local anesthetics, when the muscular dentist leaned toward the door with our pet tooth in the firm embrace of shiny forceps, we helped him to the utmost by gripping the arms of the chair with

285

Dr. Fitzgerald can be credited with the woodcut which shows the body divided into ten zones. Although Fitzgerald and Bowers discussed, in writing, the location of the reflexes on the feet there is no evidence that Fitzgerald or Dr. Bowers actually illustrated, via charts, where the reflexes appear on the feet. Dr. George Starr White, a Los Angeles physician and strong supporter of zone therapy, hints they did when he writes:

"He (Dr. Fitzgerald) discovered that the patient had either made pressures on certain parts of the hand while being operated upon, or he himself in examination had made pressure over certain areas that inhibited pain in other areas. Little by little he began to trace out these locations and systematize them."[10]

Yet, there are no illustrations in *Zone Therapy* to support the idea that Fitzgerald systematized them onto a chart of the body or on the feet.

From 1915 into the early thirties the subject of zone therapy was controversial, but did meet with a certain amount of success with doctors and dentists. Benedict Lust, M.D. in 1928 wrote, "Zone Therapy promises to become increasingly popular with drugless physicians as well as among physicians who are liberal in their ideas. In point of fact hundreds of progressive medical men all over the country are using this method at the present time, in many cases with astonishingly gratifying results."[11]

However, it cannot be said that Fitzgerald or his theories were enthusiastically received by the medical profession. As a member of the

American Medical Association, Dr. Fitzgerald first tried to teach zone therapy to his fellow physicians. It met with strong opposition from conservative physicians and those physicians who had tried the therapy without success. Fitzgerald was forced to take his knowledge to chiropractors, osteopaths, naturopaths, dentists and the public.

"One of the most disgraceful blots on the pages of organized medicine, or what is popularly known as 'The Medical Trust' is the fact that they have apparently, in every possible way, tried to hinder the spread of the gospel of Zone Therapy." claims George Starr White.[12]

One physician who did believe in Fitzgerald's work was Dr. Joe Shelby Riley of Washington D.C. Riley and his wife Elizabeth credit Dr. Fitzgerald as the one "who in modern times brought this science (zone therapy) to light."[13] Dr. Fitzgerald taught zone therapy to Dr. Riley. "Dr. Riley used this method extensively in his varied practice for many years. He probably used zone therapy more than any other single individual," write the publishers of Chesney's work, Health Research.[14] Riley was certainly one of the most untiring developers and practitioners of zone therapy. He carried the techniques out to finer points and made the first detailed diagrams and drawings of the reflex points located on the feet. He added to Fitzgerald's longitudinal zones with his discovery of eight horizontal divisions which also govern the body. His first book, *Zone Therapy Simplified* was published in 1919. During his lifetime he wrote four books in which a large portion of space was devoted to zone therapy. In addition, he wrote several correspondence courses on the subject and, in all, brought out twelve editions of his various works.

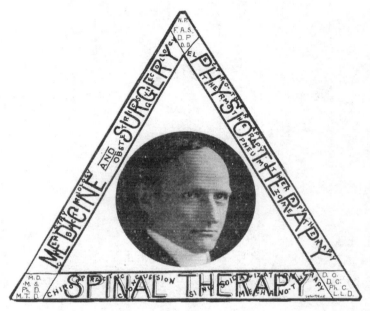

Fig. 26
Dr. Joe Shelby Riley

It should be noted that Riley's work with reflexes and zones also included the ear. Though his work had limited reflexes on the ear, it is the earliest Western record of including the ears in zone therapy. Auriculotherapy, as ear reflexology is termed, was also practiced by the Chinese through the ages. A French doctor, Paul Nogier brought ear reflexes again to the attention of the West in the 1950's. Today, Director of the American Academy of Reflexol-

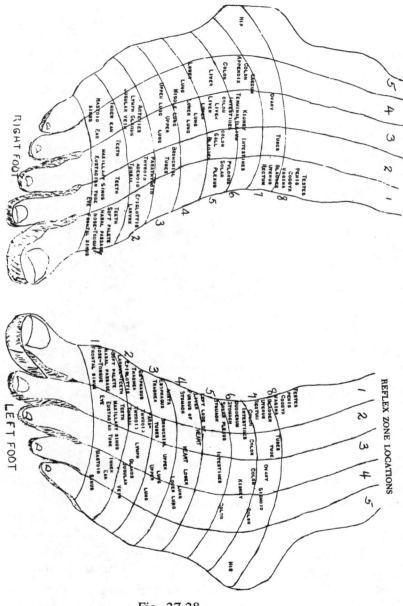

Fig. 27-28
Foot charts by Dr. Joe Shelby Riley

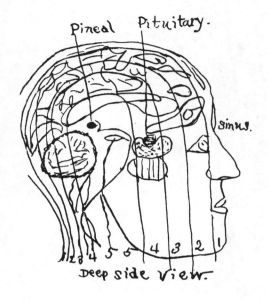

Deep side view.

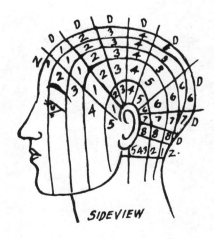

SIDEVIEW

Fig. 29-30
Head charts by Dr. Joe Shelby Riley

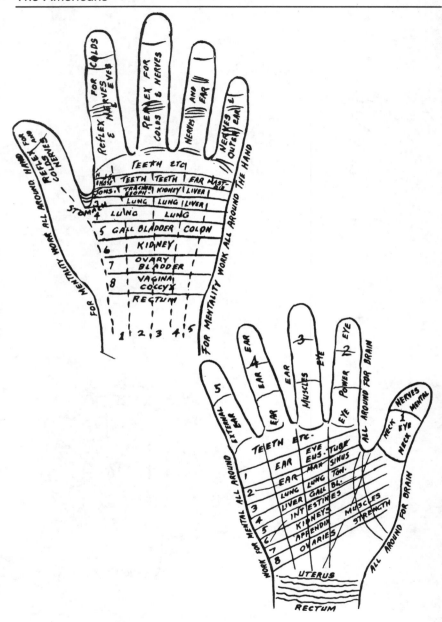

Fig. 31-32
Hand charts by Dr. Joe Shelby Riley

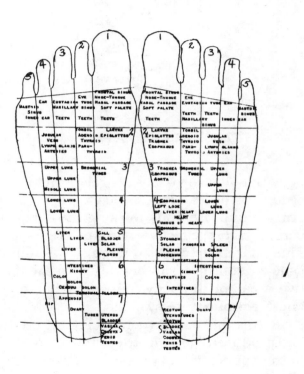

Fig. 33
Foot chart by Dr. Joe Shelby Riley

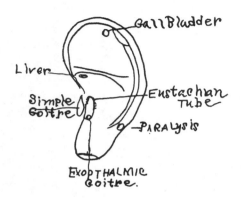

Fig. 34
Ear chart by Dr. Joe Shelby Riley

ogy, Bill Flocco of Los Angeles includes the study of the ear reflexes as part of his core curriculum. He finds working the ear reflexes can be most effective with problems of the muscular system. In addition, Dr. Ralph Alan Dale covers the ear in his works on the reiterative areas of the body found in what he calls Micro-acupuncture systems.

Returning to zone therapy, Fitzgerald's work had produced "non-electrical applicators" to aid in the application of pressure. These included aluminum combs and bands, ordinary surgical clamps, a nasal probe, and a metal tongue depressor among other things. The use of rubber bands and wooden spring clothes pins was also employed. Riley eliminated the clothes pins, rubber bands and other gadgets and developed a "hooking" technique.[15]

Riley was a well educated man of many interests. His studies included medicine, surgery, physio-therapy, chiropractics, zone therapy, osteopathy, naturopathy, electro-therapy, color and light therapy, as well as an interest in the occult. The Rileys ran a school in Washington D.C. with a curriculum which encompassed most of the above therapies while they continued to find time to treat private patients. To escape the harsh winters of the Northeast they wintered in Florida.

During the early 1930's Eunice Ingham (1879-1974) worked with Dr. Riley as his therapist in St. Petersburg, Florida. Her contribution to reflexology has been profound. She was a real pioneer who was determined to help people help themselves if their doctor was not interested in using reflexology. Ingham separated work on the reflexes of the feet from zone therapy in general, although she continued to use the term. Later she called her work "compression massage" and finally settled on the use of the word "reflexology". Reports Dwight Byers, her nephew, "In the early years she worked with doctors to prove her findings, and to prove to them that reflexology was a useful diagnostic tool. My aunt lectured at a medical clinic headed by Dr. Charles Epstein in May 1939. In his report he acknowledged reflexology worked. While they knew it worked, doctors weren't interested in using it because reflexology was too time consuming. They couldn't make as much money."[16]

Eunice made two major contributions. Her first was that she found an alternating pres-

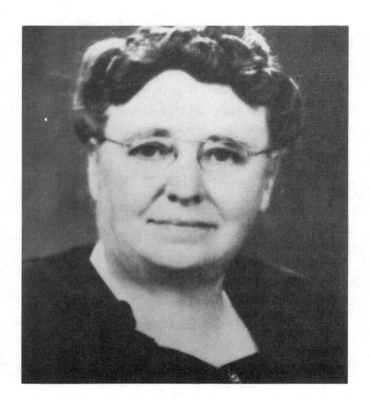

Fig. 35
Eunice Ingham, Mother of Modern Reflexology

sure, rather than having a numbing effect, stimulated healing. One early technique Ingham used was to tape wads of cotton over tender spots on the feet. The theory being that the client could continue to stimulate the reflexes and hurry the healing process along as he or she walked about. Though the clients got better Ingham soon discarded this technique when she realized this over stimulated the reflexes which brought about some reactions.[17]

Secondly, with encouragement from Riley[18] and other drugless doctors, she took her work to the public and the non-medical community. Though they could not use her method to diagnose, prescribe or treat for a specific illness, Ingham realized that lay people could learn the proper reflexology techniques to help themselves, their families and friends. Over the years Eunice was called upon by the drugless community to speak at conventions. She shared her techniques and knowledge with chiropodists, massage and pyhsiotherapists, naturopaths and osteopaths.

In 1938 her research resulted in the book *Stories the Feet Can Tell.* With the publication of her book Ingham traveled up and down the East Coast giving seminars. She went on to write three more books: *Zone Therapy and Gland Reflexes*, in 1945 which was later revised, enlarged and printed as *Stories the Feet Have Told* in 1951. In the early 60's she wrote *Stories the Feet Are Telling* which was never published. According to Byers this book contained her seminar syllabus.

In the different editions of her books, Eunice Ingham switches the use of the terms "zone therapy", "compression massage" and "reflexology" back and forth. "It did take her years to finally settle on the use of the word reflexology," notes Byers. "Eunice mingled the terms and changed them depending on how things were going at the time of publication. She was always afraid of getting into trouble with the American Medical Association. She tried to stay away from medical sounding words, so she couldn't be persecuted for practicing medicine without a license. For years she would only have 100 or 200 copies made per printing. My aunt didn't want a large number around to be confiscated by the authorities. That would have meant a great loss of money to her since she self-published," states Byers.[19] In addition to her fear of legal reprisals, Eunice switched from the use of the words "zone therapy" to describe her work to "compression massage" for more practical reasons. She did not use gadgets as most zone therapists did and she also restricted her work to the feet. She did not want her method confused with massage either. Eventually she omitted the use of the term 'compression massage' too.

The years of World War II ended Ingham's traveling for a time. She spent the interim writing *Zone Therapy and Gland Reflexes*. Ingham quotes an interesting story from an unusual source in the book. The November 1944 issue of *Hospital Corps Quarterly* published by the Department of the Navy, Medicine and Surgery, ran an article about zone physio-therapy. The piece tells the story of B.S. Shope, PhM2c, stationed at Camp Pendleton who cured the 13-day hiccough spell experienced by an aircraft worker in Los Angeles. Shope massaged the man's feet for an hour, explaining that massaging the nerve reflexes was soothing and relaxing. An earlier curing of hiccough by

Shope, using the same technique, had also been reported in the local papers.[20]

In 1942, at 53, Eunice married for the first time. Her husband was Fred Stopfel, a widowed client whom she had helped overcome a problem with asthma. When gas rationing ended in 1946, she and Fred struck out for the West Coast. "They were a great pair," says Byers. "With Fred's help they could drive west and had the freedom to stop and give seminars along the way," continued Byers. Dwight Byers and his sister Eusebia Messenger, R.N. joined their aunt's lecture circuit in 1947.

Each of Eunice's seminars was unique. Her method of instruction was to demonstrate and lecture as she worked on the health problems of those who attended. Over the years Byers contributed to Ingham's work by better organizing the seminar presentation into a standard format, while Eusebia endeavored to make the charts more anatomically correct. The written work, however, continued to be Eunice's alone and she modified or updated her books at each publishing. The one exception to anatomy which Eunice made was her insistence that the reflex to the heart be located in the third and fourth zone. Anatomically the heart is located on the midline of the body, therefore to be anatomically correct the heart reflex should be located on the big toe side of the foot. Instead Eunice found she got the best results when she worked the heart reflex on the bottom of the left foot beneath the fourth and fifth toes.

Eunice criss-crossed the country for over thirty years as she taught her method through books, charts and seminars to thousands of people in and out of the medical profession.

Though Ingham was promoting self-help, her students, who used reflexology professionally began coming under attack for practicing medicine without a license in the 1950's. Several private letters to Eunice bear this out. In 1955 The State of Nebraska's Department of Health referred to reflexology as quackery and its practice was against the law. The Board of Medical and Osteopathic Examiners of South Dakota took a stand against reflexology in 1956.[21] In Buffalo, New York Mrs. Ann Burzynski, a licensed masseuse, was charged by the State Education Department of practicing medicine without a license. However, the City Court jury deliberated only a few minutes before acquitting her.[22]

In a similar case, a jury of eight men and four women found Anna Mazzarelli from Encino, California not guilty of the same charge in January 1961. The case was brought against Mrs. Mazzarelli by the State Board of Medical Examiners who contended, "Mrs. Mazzarelli claimed to cure everything from liver ailments to mental retardation by massaging the nerve ending in the toes." Recounts Mazzarelli, "I was charged and summoned to appear in court for practicing medicine without a license. My mother had died the month before. Thank God! She would have been so ashamed. My attorney advised me to plead 'no contest', pay the fine and get on with my life. I refused, because that would be admitting guilt and I was innocent. So against his advice I decided to fight my case in court. I did demand two things: 1) that I have a jury trial; and 2) that I be allowed to give a treatment in court during the trial so the jury could see for themselves what I do."[23] Mazzarelli's defense pointed out that she was a licensed cosmetologist and as such was entitled to give massages and other similar treatments. As the week long trial proceeded, Mazzarelli actually did demonstrate her techniques on a woman spectator.

Mazzarelli was questioned by both the judge and the city attorney. In response to the question from the city attorney: "If you wanted to cure a liver disability, you would massage the little toe. Is that right?" she replied, "I massage the body as a unit." The attorney continued, "If someone came to you with a stomach problem, would you massage his feet?" To which she answered, "I'd refer him to a doctor."[24]

"Eunice came out, by train, from the East and was willing to testify for me. She had read about my case in the paper back there. I never asked her to come or to testify, she just volunteered to do it. But, she wasn't called to testify." said Anna.

Eunice would face her own court case in 1968. The State of New York charged her with practicing medicine without a license that year, but dropped the charges before the case went to court. Two years later Eunice, at 81, "retired" from the lecture circuit. She died in 1974, after devoting forty years of her life to reflexology. Today, her legacy continues under the direction of Byers.

The International Institute of Reflexology in St. Petersburg, Florida, directed by Byers, has continued to grow as it has expanded its educational program to present seminars in Europe, South Africa, New Zealand, Australia as well as across the United States and Canada. Most authors on reflexology including, Hanne Marquardt in Germany, Doreen Bayly of England, Barbara and Kevin Kunz, Mildred Carter, Laura Norman, and Anna Kaye all of the U.S., to name only a few, have at one time studied the Ingham method.

Practiced by people both professionally or on relatives and friends, reflexology continues to gain momentum. Over the years, information about reflexology has been available from two main sources: through the Ingham/Byers seminars, and the efforts of Health Research Publishing of Mokelumne Hill, California. Health Research publishes reprints of the earliest works on zone therapy authored by Fitzgerald, Riley and others. In the 1960's Prentice-Hall was the first major publisher of new works on reflexology. They began with Mildred Carter's book, *Helping Yourself with Foot Reflexology*. With sales of 500,000 copies, Carter has brought reflexology greater recognition. Her book actually blazed the path for the proliferation of self-help books on the market today. This was not done without a fight, however. In *Whole Life Monthly* Carter shared the story of her fight with the American Medical Association.

"After my first book was published, a pudgy man from the AMA showed up at my house and

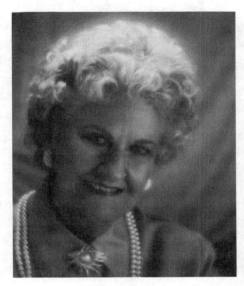

Fig. 36
Mildred Carter

ranted and raved for about twenty minutes and viciously warned me never to practice again and never to write another book on Reflexology. He stormed away and shortly thereafter, the AMA sued Prentice-Hall for printing such a book."[25]

Further explains Carter, "I was naive, but protected, when my book was published. I let Prentice-Hall put the copyright in their name instead of mine. The AMA thought I wouldn't have the money to fight them and it would be an easy case to win. But instead of me they had to sue Prentice-Hall because they held the copyright. Prentice-Hall had lots of money to hire good lawyers. There was a court trial and Prentice-Hall won the right to continue publication after presenting hundreds of letters from my readers in court as part of our defense. The point was, I wasn't trying to practice medicine without a license."

The AMA continued to watch Carter closely. Later she received another visit by the same man. This time the representative of the AMA carried with him a letter Mrs. Carter had written to a woman in response to one she received about the woman's daughter who was in a coma. Continues Carter:

"Doctors had told her there was no hope for the child and that she should just be put in a rest home. I wrote her a letter telling her not to believe the doctors and that this black cloud was blocking the healing forces of light. At the end of the letter I told her that I was a Reflexologist and if she wanted to speak, I would gladly talk with her. And then I signed it...Well, anyway, the AMA representative just glared and glared at me and began stomping around my living room screaming, 'We got you this time ol' girl. We're going to put you in the penitentiary!' Finally when he was done screaming I told him I didn't think people would approve of the AMA sending a woman to prison for doing her life's work. I then told him I was a Minister and he just about jumped out of his skin. I then went and got my certificate and handed it to him. Now, when he took the certificate his eyes seemed to bulge and he started shaking all over...I really thought I'd have to give him a reflexology treatment to save his life!"[26]

As reflexology has gained wider recognition with the public there are many books available on the subject which teach both theory and practical techniques. Before looking more closely at the scientific basis of reflexology we will quickly look at the practice of reflexology today and how it is used around the world.

CHAPTER 4

REFLEXOLOGY TODAY

*T*en years ago Noelle Weyeneth, president of the Swiss Reflexology Association spent three weeks in jail for practicing reflexology. Today, the Swiss government is funding a reflexology research study. How times have changed.

Recent interest in complementary health practices around the globe which began in the 1980's has brought greater focus on reflexology. It is the role of reflexology to help and it should be thought of as a complementary therapy rather than an alternative therapy. The use of the term alternative implies that reflexology is better than something else or should be used in place of some other therapy. It sets the reflexologist up as being in competition with other modalities and conventional medicine. There is no need to challenge other modalities as reflexology used as a stress reduction technique is generally a complement to any other form of treatment employed.

Both those in and out of mainstream medicine are finding reflexology helpful. Athletes are using reflexology to enhance performance and speed the healing of injuries as well as to relieve pain due to injury or overwork. New York Ranger hockey player Ron Greschner credits reflexology with getting him back on the ice. Greschner's back kept him sidelined most of the 1982-83 season. When he began seeing a reflexologist his back slowly mended. "I don't know what happened medically," Greschner says. "I haven't had a back X-ray since 1983. All I know is that I've been hit hard, and I can lift rocks on our farm in up-state New York, and it doesn't bother me," he explains. [1]

Reflexologists have participated in "demonstration" booths at the California Police Olympics since the summer of 1985 introducing athletes and their families to reflexology. A San Francisco Bay Area police athletic director was so impressed he plans to incorporate reflexology into the training practice of his men to relax their strained muscles. Many athletes feel reflexology gives them the competitive edge. One example of this is George Cohen. Cohen works for the Los Angeles Department of Corrections as a parole officer. In 1987 he won three gold medals in the track and field events, and credited reflexology with contributing heavily to his success.

Ted Cooke, Chief of Police in Culver City, California feels the same way. In a letter thanking Jerry Budenz, who coordinated the presence of reflexologists at the event, he wrote, "I won the gold medal in racquetball. I did this, I think, because following the workout which you and your associates gave my feet I felt completely rejuvenated and fresh. I intend to do this each time I compete."[2]

During the 1987 games a small informal blood pressure study was conducted by the Sacramento Valley Reflexology Association. It was found that reflexology normalized (either bringing it up or down as needed) the systolic pressure in seventy-five percent the cases and the diastolic pressure in sixty-one percent of those cases studied.[3]

The same techniques can also be used successfully in medical cases. Eleven years ago Directors Ruth Hahn and Gloria Hufford of The Rehabilitation Center for Neurological Development in Piqua, Ohio added reflexology to the Center's program of sensory-motor exercises. Because forty percent of brain input pathways is through tactile sensation they have found that deep foot massage with a nylon brush stimulates the autonomic nervous system that controls various body protective functions. The Center continues to document the use of traditional reflexology too. It has been found that reflexology relaxes the rigidity of the foot in the brain injured. Reflexology Research Project, directed by the Kunzes, has experienced much the same results with their work on paralysis clients.

Nurses in Switzerland have found that using reflexology on terminally ill cancer patients does not stop the cancer or death but it does make the patients more comfortable. Reflexology improves the quality of life and leads to a more dignified death. Writes Barbara Zeller Dobbs of the Geneva School of Nursing, "Our purpose for using reflexology with these patients (terminally ill with cancer) was to decrease their pain but we soon realized the beneficial effect of reflexology on the morale of patients and families. Patients expressed feelings of being less abandoned and the families expressed satisfaction at seeing that something painless existed that could aid their relative."[4]

Reflexologist Larry Clemmons of Chicago agrees that reflexology can be an "useful tool" in controlling pain. He believes that stimulating a painful reflex point on the foot sends signals to the brain that, when needed, stimulates the production of the body's pain suppressing chemicals called endorphins. This interrupts the pain cycle, eases pain and helps the body to relax.[5]

Although the American Medical Association does not recognize reflexology, several physicians across the United States do believe in the use of reflexology for stress and pain reduction. Dr. Susan Wright of Chicago's Rush Medical Center is a pain management specialist who recommends reflexology along with other non-traditional modalities such as acupressure, shiatsu, biofeedback, self hypnosis, massage and imagery to fight the pain of arthritis.[6] Louise Lockard, M.D. a family practitioner from Denver sends some of her patients to reflexologist Zachary Brinkerhoff as an alternative treatment for stress. "Many of my patients have problems that I can [only] partially treat so I send them to people like Mr. Brinkerhoff," Lockard says. "I'm still deciding how to fit it in with my conventional understanding," she concludes.[7]

Dr. Ray Wunderlick of St. Petersburg, Florida is quoted as saying, "Reflexology is most helpful in persons who have painful conditions of the body, who have hypertension, anxiety and difficulty in tuning their bodies down." If one had to choose between tranquilizers and reflexology Wunderlick says he would, "take reflexology every time. The side effects are minimal and there's no question that it's a safe way to induce relaxation."[8]

Bernie Siegel, a Yale-New Haven Hospital surgeon who works frequently with terminal cancer patients endorses reflexology too. He describes it as "a total healing experience for the whole person." Vera Zablozki, M.D. concurs. She writes, "As a medical doctor specializing in neurology, and from both my medical knowledge and my personal experience, I can only give my full approval to this old-new method. I hope that more physicians will accept reflexology as part of their standard treatment modality."[9]

The use of reflexology is worldwide. It is being used in a fertility clinic in Argentina, in drug dependency and alcohol rehabilitation centers in the U.S., in reflex therapy clinics in Russia, in hospitals in Germany and elsewhere in Europe, and as a low cost health care system in the Philippines and underdeveloped countries.[10] Reflexology is a simple discipline requiring no expensive, hi-tech equipment. This is probably one of the reasons there is universal interest in reflexology.

Even Hollywood script writers have discovered reflexology to be good subject material. During the 1988 season, reflexology was used as part of a plot or referred to in fifteen different prime time television shows! At the same time numerous magazines ranging from *Playboy* to chiropractic journals to women and health magazines have reported on the subject.[11]

Reflexologist themselves are getting together. In late November 1987, The Philippine Association of Natural Holistic Health Professionals, Inc. held its first national convention in Manila. The event was warmly greeted by such dignitaries as President Corazon Aquino, The Archbishop of Manila, and the Secretary of Health. Alfredo R.A. Bengzon M.D., Secretary of Health said in his message to the convention, "The practice of Reflexology should be interwoven with the concept of primary health care to attain good health and self reliance. I fervently wish that your organization, new officers and members will continue in the pursuit of providing equal opportunity to our less privilege countrymen to enjoy good health."

Dr. Manubay, president of the Association and the founder of AKSEM Holistic Reflexology in the Philippines, who studied the Ingham method in the United States, says he has graduated thousands of professionals through his program. Kaye Wade, a stuntwoman and reflexologist from Studio City, California was in the Philippines to shoot a movie during the spring of 1988. When her shooting schedule permitted, she travelled to Manila for a session at the AKSEM Center. Kay reports, "the reflexologists at the Center were pleasant, honest and knowledgeable about health. They were enthused about reflexology and acupressure; really believing in the benefits of both." Reflexology is respected and taken seriously in the Philippines, both by the public and the practitioner. Kay continued, "Part of Dr. Manubay's training includes 30 hours of community work—that is going out to housing projects to work on the sick and elderly."[12]

Reflexologists met in Piqua, Ohio, outside of Dayton, for a research conference October 15-16, 1989. Research reports included topics as diverse as reflexology being used with chemical dependency programs, to it being used with the brain injured. A tour of the Rehabilitation Center for Neurological Development where reflexology has been used as part of the Center's sensory-motor exercise program was part of the conference.

As Ruth Hahn led a tour of the facility she related the story of how the Center came to be and why the application of reflexology is important to the brain injured. "We all feel there are pieces of a puzzle that need to be put together to help the brain injured improve. So far we have uncovered six puzzle pieces. These include: 1) neurological development; 2) nutrition; 3) vitamin and herb supplements; 4) foot reflexology; 5) educational kinesiology; and 6) cranial osteopathy," shared Ruth.

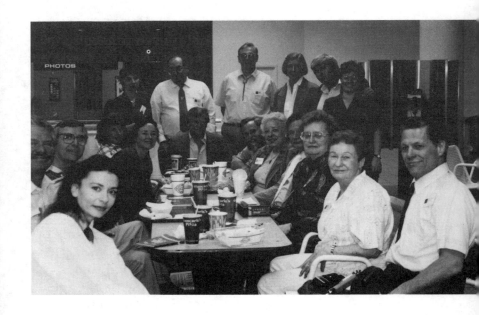

Fig. 37
October 1989 RRP/CNAR Research Conference, Piqua
Ohio. l. to r. Seated, Maria Brinkerhoff-Denver CO,
Bill Runquist-Jackson CA, Tom Gardiner-Mt. Clemens
MI, Laura Norman-NYC, Barbara Mosier-Littleton
CO, Joseph Horan-NYC, Joel Swartz-Rochester NY,
Mary Lou & Bill Vanderlaan-Crown Point IN, Irene
Melnyk-Winnepeg, Manitoba, Ruby Bisson-New
Liskeard, Ontario, Zachary Brinkerhoff-Denver CO.
Standing l. to r. Christine Issel-Sacramento CA, Jerry
Budenz-Camarillo CA, Bob Dooley-Ft. Madison IA,
Barbara & Kevin Kunz-Albuquerque NM, Josephine
Tan, Singapore. Not pictured, Pat Covault-Ft. Wayne
IN.

Interest in the conference came from Athens and South Africa as well as across Canada and the United States. One of the participants, Josephine Tan came from Singapore to attend.

In North America reflexologists are striving towards professionalism. The first Conference of North American Reflexologists (CNAR) was held in Denver, May 27-28, 1989. The format for this conference was preceded by one in Los Angeles for California reflexologists held March 3-4, 1989.

The California conference, aided by the Schneider Report[13] began with a look at professionalism and what it takes to be a profession. According to Schneider there is a branch of sociology devoted to the study of professionalism. In 1957, sociologist Earnest Greenwood isolated five traits of professions that other sociologists agreed were indicators of a profession, and that either were not found in occupations classified as non-professional, or not present to the same degree. These five points were:

1) A systematic theory or body of knowledge;

2) Authority—others look up to the professional and suspend their own judgement;

3) Community sanction—the public is convinced of the importance and need for the profession to be practiced;

4) Has established an ethical code of conduct; and

5) Has a culture composed of norms, symbols and values.

Norms are the social interaction which exists between the professional and the client;

and between the professionals themselves. Symbols are the things that carry meaning both to the public and to the professional—examples include, an insignia or logo, special vocabulary, or dress that sets the profession apart and is easily identifiable to the profession (this would include things like the foot and hand charts),

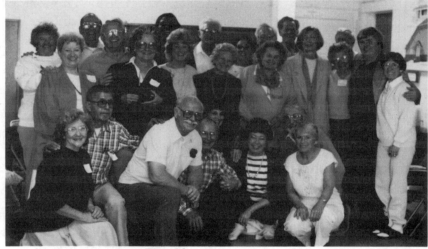

Fig. 38
March 1989 California Conference of Reflexologists, Los Angeles, California. First row kneeling l. to r: Betty Heyman, Larry Kaneshiro, Ron Wilbanks, Andy Bukowitz, Christine Issel, Muff Warren, Norm Secker, Lisa Long. Second, standing l. to r: Ann Ferro, Howard Wylie, Margaret Orosz, Bobbi Warren, Mildred Carter, Oma Teuwen, Barbara Kunz, Frances Alonge, Kevin Kunz, Toni Wilbanks. Third row l. to r: Roberta White, Jerry Budenz, Sylvia Quarles, Jim Ingram, Gwen Barnett, Walt Gosting, Bill Wilson, Warren Pierpoint. Not pictured: Hannah Stein, Mary Ann Blancarte, Freya Alexander, David Allan and Tino Zandredino.

and has a unique history. Values are a field's belief that the service rendered is for the community good , and the community would suffer without it. In addition, the professionals know more than the non-professionals; their knowledge can further social progress; and through rationality and attention to objectivity, knowledge will expand and be accepted only with proof.

Kevin Kunz reminded those assembled that, "Credibility for the study and professional practice of reflexology can be created by the profession. Just as with any profession which formalizes its practices, additional responsibilities are assumed by the profession. Responsibilities are taken to define the acceptable level of practice by the practitioner and to provide a public perception of a service which is safe, legal, beneficial and well performed. The study and the responsibility to define, defend and further the study are a part of the professional as well."

In California the following general subjects were explored: 1) professional development—establishing ways to shape our own destiny and not become regulated by governmental authorities or under some other profession; 2) develop a unified professional organization; 3) establish a state-wide educational policy which defines training requirements; 4) scientific research and development; and 5) agree on a universal definition. The goals that were set for the definition were: a) to be generic; b) something which could be taken to city hall when applying for a business license; c) expresses why reflexology is different than massage; and d) something which a practitioner could individualize by adding his own sentence to the end.

Forming a definition was strenuous, time consuming and the cause of much debate. In the conference brochure for the California Conference of Reflexology, Bill Flocco, owner and director of The American Academy of Reflexology warned, "Caution should be taken not to limit the definition of reflexology. Discussions made now can confine or leave vistas open in the future should legislation with resultant advantages and disadvantages result."[14]

The California definition agreed upon was: "Foot and hand reflexology is the physical act of applying pressure to the reflex areas and zones in the feet and hands with specific thumb, finger and hand techniques performed without oils, lotions or creams; with the premise that a physiological change can take place in the body."[15]

Supporters of the Council of North American Reflexologists conference in Denver included four authors, five schools/or methodologies, three associations, two countries, a dozen states and two provinces. This was the first time reflexologists from different schools and countries had gotten together in North America with the idea of working together for the advancement of reflexology as a profession. In Denver a similar approach as that taken in California was used. In the end all participants agreed on five points. These included the need: 1) to form an umbrella association; 2) to develop a certification program; 3) to create a universal definition; 4) to establish professional standards and practices; and 5) to form a legal coalition.[16] Those who attended the conference agreed to continue to work together on the issues above which are currently under study and other areas of concern.

In Denver, the concepts for the definition were the same, but the wording was different. "Foot and hand reflexology is based on the premise that there are zones and reflex areas in the feet and hands which correspond to all body parts. The physical act of applying specific pressures using thumb, finger and hand techniques performed without oils, lotions or creams results in stress reduction causing a physiological change in the body."[17]

The debate is far from over. Further discussions most certainly will take place before a universal definition is finalized.

The need for a legal coalition was in response to the latest threat to reflexology. The State of Florida's Department of Professional Regulation (DPR) passed, in 1987, a new ruling. In Florida it is considered a misconduct and negligence to engage in the practice of reflexology without a current massage license. The Department of Professional Regulation does not accept reflexology as a separate modality and has lumped it with massage which makes reflexologists subject to rule by the massage community. Reflexologists are no longer in control of their own field! "By doing this DPR is saying all body work techniques come from the five basic massage techniques. We have a history to debate that. Even our tradition is different," argues Kevin Kunz.[18] "We want our books (books on reflexology) and our body of knowledge to represent the industry. Massage schools certainly don't use a massage book to teach reflexology, so why should we pass a massage license to practice?" questions Kunz. In defining reflexology, DPR, in essence, took the definition of massage, changed a few words and now uses it to define reflexology. Kunz feels

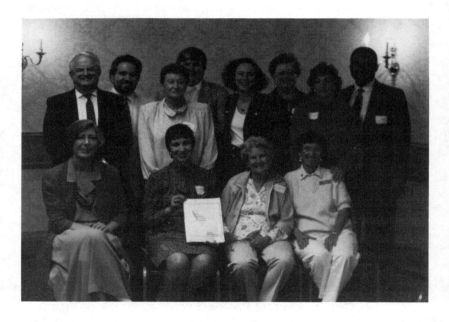

Fig. 39
May 1989 Conference of North American
Reflexologists, Denver, Colorado. Seated l. to r:
Barbara Kunz, Christine Issel, Mildred Carter, Toni
Wilbanks. Standing l. to r: Howard Wylie, George
Balut, Ruby Bisson, Kevin Kunz, Laura Norman, Irene
Melnyk, Barbara Mosier, Larry Clemmons.

we need to challenge this by questioning their source material through a legal coalition.

Legal problems for reflexologists did not end in the sixties after the charges against Eunice Ingham were dropped. Over the years cases have been rumored in Ohio, Oregon, Indiana, and California. In 1982, Judy Turner, working in Illinois, was found guilty of practicing medicine and podiatry without a license. Turner fought for over a year and was convicted of: 1) diagnosing using reflexology because foot charts hung on the wall; and 2) prescribing because she offered for sale and recommended a bottle of aloe vera juice, saying it was good for general health. Turner was fined $650.[19]

Jay Skiles of Crescent City, California was told reflexology was illegal in the State of California and therefore he was denied the economic opportunity of participating in a health fair. He reported his situation to the Kunzes. Through their attorney Barbara and Kevin Kunz challenged the Board of Medical Quality Assurance ruling in California. In a letter from Linda McCready, coordinator for the Division of Allied Health Professions, to John Myers, attorney for the Kunzes she wrote, "Under current law, California does not license the practice of reflexology. Since there is no section of law waiving licensure or permitting its unlicensed practice, and since the practice of massage AS A TREATMENT is included in the scopes of practice for specific professions, by extension it is unlawful for an unlicensed person to practice reflexology in this state."

"Non-therapeutic massage for purposes of relaxation or recreation is not affected by these laws so long as the practitioner does not make any representations to clients that it constitutes treatment or that a condition exists which would be affected by massage." ended McCready.[20]

In essence a reflexologist cannot practice reflexology for health benefits! However, he may legally practice it for relaxation purposes.

It appears that throughout the United States reflexologists are either required—usually not by the state but by local municipalities—to have a massage license, which is designed as an anti-prostitution measure, or an occupational license in addition to a business license. A reflexologist who practices in more than one locale, that is under a different jurisdiction, must then have a license to practice in that area also. This can be very expensive if a reflexologist works on an out-call basis, seeing clients in their homes in several different communities.

Monday, April 12, 1993 marked a milestone in reflexology history. At 12:08 P.M. North Dakota Governor Edward Schafer signed a bill which established the first reflexology board in the country. The legislative battle started in 1990 when amendments to the existing state wide massage law were to go into effect. The North Dakota Massage Therapy Association (NDMTA), the state chapter of the American Massage Therapy Association (AMTA) in 1989 successfully passed a bill that would have required anyone practicing acupressure, reflexology and polarity to become a registered massage therapist by December 29, 1990. According to a letter written by Mary Muehlen Maring counsel for the NDMTA to comply would have meant that reflexologists needed to "present a diploma or credentials issued by a school of massage approved by the AMTA or show that they were an active member of AMTA." In addition, they needed "to pass a reasonable demonstrative, oral and written examination conducted by the Board in the art of body massage."

Under the leadership of Arlene McHenry, a North Dakota Reflexology Association was founded in January of 1991 with McHenry acting as president. The group began the legislative process of getting reflexology exempt from the law. The legislature gave them two years to prepare legislation for their own board at the next legislative session.

Working with Senator John Traynor and NDRA members Christine Issel invested untold hours writing the law and spent time in North Dakota testifying before the House and Senate committees in 1990 and 1992 in order to help NDRA achieve its hard earned success. Bill Flocco, who was a veteran professional lobbyist, before becoming a reflexologist acted as consultant to Issel. Others involved in the letter writing campaigns to the legislature included Larry Clemmons, Dwight Byers, Marcia Aschendorf, Kevin Kunz, Billie Scott, Bill Runquist and Dr. Harvey Lampell.

Flocco cautioned, "What worked in North Dakota will not work in the same way in any other state. Every state has its own individual legislative and political dynamics. Individual differences in each state must be honored. If not, the results could be the opposite of the success in North Dakota."

While North Dakota has the distinction of being the first state with its own reflexology board, reflexologists in other states are also working to protect the right of reflexologists to practice as a separate discipline. Exemptions for reflexologists from state massage laws are in effect in Maine and New Mexico. In 1990 thanks largely to the work of Janet Stetser, reflexology was excluded from the massage registration law. Due to the work of Kevin and Barbara Kunz reflexology gained an exemption in New Mexico as a native healing method. In California, reflexologists are part of the California Coalition of Somatic Practices, which is a group looking into legislative options that would include all modalities.

During the CNAR conference in Denver, Larry Clemmons, of Chicago, expressed his concern for the survival of reflexology as a separate profession. "One of the things clear to me is the necessity of having some kind of national standard that says: This is what reflexology is, this is what is agreed to by reflexologists across the country as a *minimum* standard of practice and behavior. This national standard would be the traditional body of knowledge that defines and describes, within a limited range, what reflexology is and the techniques that constitute reflexology. This doesn't mean you cannot do something in addition to the techniques agreed upon. I'm saying there must be some standards to which other associations and professions can point and know that this is what the term reflexology means. We need to set the tone now to define and improve our image, or some other profession will take us over," Clemmons said as he addressed those assembled.[21]

There is little doubt that if reflexology is going to be a self-regulated system it needs to establish several vehicles. One agency is a licensing board whose primary concern is protection of the public. A licensing board or credentialing agency assures the public of the competency of the practitioner and provides a certificate to the reflexologists to that effect. The reflexologist, in turn, would need to meet certain professional and ethical standards in their practice. This would include full and fair disclosure of services and training to the consumer.

To meet this need, Clemmons working with others, late in 1990, founded a nonprofit corporation called the American Reflexology Certification Board (ARCB). National certification with ARCB is a voluntary process by which a nongovernmental organization recognizes an individual who has met certain qualifications of knowledge and skill within the field regardless of which method or school he attended. While national certification distinguishes one as a qualified professional, it still leaves the person who is not certified free to practice without penalty.

A second vehicle is a professional membership association whose goals involve the advancement of the members' interest. This body would provide the profession continuing education or special interest seminars and conferences beyond basic education, public relations, and would lobby governmental authorities.

In the past few years many new statewide reflexology associations have been formed. As these organizations communicate with each other some type of national association will no doubt emerge.

It is important and necessary that both agencies remain separate and distinct because goal confusion leads to conflict of interest and destroys the integrity and validity of the credential. Both organizations must also be open to all reflexologists regardless of methodology learned or employed.

Reflexology in the United States, with these two vehicles, could become a self-regulatory system proclaiming its professional standards and practices to others.

On an international scale, September 29, 1990 saw the inauguration of the International Council of Reflexologists (ICR) at a conference held in Toronto which was jointly sponsored by the Reflexology Association of Canada and the Council of North American Reflexologists. The ICR charter reflects the thinking of many minds and was drawn up using the United Nations charter as a guideline. Due to different national laws governing each country and even within sections of a country, the decisions of the ICR General Council will be merely recommendations and are not legally binding. However, based on the principle of voluntary association, members of ICR commit themselves to act in pursuance of ICR purposes and in conformity with its principles for the development of reflexology as a profession.

The ICR is conceived as a multipurpose organization designed to lend credibility and legitimacy to the field of reflexology. ICR is committed to meeting the needs of the profession by conducting a biennial conference, providing a forum for the exchange of ideas and information, and by supporting local, regional and national associations.

How reflexology will develop in the future is anybody's guess. But judging from the response of reflexologists they are committed to creating the future of reflexology today. Kevin Kunz opened the ICR conference in Toronto by saying we are entering into the Golden Age of Reflexology. Speaker after speaker brought something unique to the program. We learned about the early days of reflexology with Dwight Byers as he spoke of his aunt Eunice Ingham, and Mildred Carter related her experience with the AMA. May Post, Joel Swartz and Zachary Brinkerhoff gave us food for thought as they presented new ideas and techniques. Psychologist Tom Gardiner shared a possible new use for reflexology. He has found it a very useful tool in his practice as he helps those dealing with chemical dependency and drug addiction. Gardiner says it eases withdrawal symptoms and helps the patient stay clean. Dr. Simon Wikler, a podiatrist from Florida explained why he thinks every cardiologist should have a reflexologist on staff and the future he sees for reflexology in the medical field. He talked about shoe related diseases and specific exercises to combat them which can be easily incorporated into our current methods of doing reflexology.[22]

During subsequent conferences in Virginia Beach, Virginia USA in 1991 and Kos, Greece in 1992 ICR has gained global momentum with eighteen different countries participating. Speakers have shared the legal status of reflexology in their country as well as educational standards. Some of the foremost leaders of reflexology on a global scale have acted as guest lecturers educating those who attended in new theories and methods. Other countries around the world are also beginning to hold their own national conferences and to run research studies. These activities are critical to the universal growth of reflexology.

Reflexology is the wave of the future according to marketing forecaster Irma Zendl. In a recent newspaper article Zendl, who at forty, earns $400,000 annually predicting trends for such companies as Procter and Gamble, Reebok, McDonalds, and Pepsi spots the next big trend as foot reflexology.[23] The question is will the profession be able to remain autonomous and meet the demand for qualified practitioners. It is certain that the field has a rich history, different traditions, and a body of knowledge separate from any other profession. For the benefit of the public, reflexology needs to remain a separate modality. It appears that today's reflexologists around the world are doing their share by actively working to create their own future.

SECTION II

**The
Science of
Reflexology**

Start a new chapter

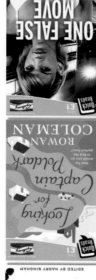

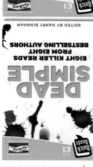

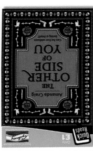
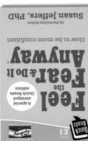
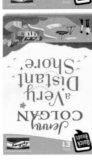
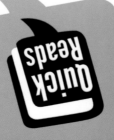

CHAPTER 5

REFLEXOLOGY THEORIES

*I*t is impossible to apply strictly rational empirical criteria to determine how reflexology works, because like any therapy there is an art side to its application. The relationship between the client and practitioner can alter results. Also, there can be no ultimate explanation for the workings of the human body and the possibilities of help are endless because the body sometimes responds in unexpected ways. The dynamics of reflexology embraces all systems of the body: the nervous system, muscles, blood, lymph, and all the organs. To understand how and why reflexology works, again following the trail from a historical perspective, the theories put forth over the years by various authors will be examined before we look at scientific research.

Dr. Fitzgerald did not use the term "reflex" in his work. He contended, however, that the human body has independent nerve zones, and that pressure upon the centers controlling these areas affects abnormal conditions in every part of the particular zone. In *Zone Therapy* by Fitzgerald and Bowers, four reasons are given for the way zone therapy works:

1) (through) the soothing influence of animal magnetism;

2) the manipulation of the hand over the injured place tends to prevent a condition of venous statis (bruising);

3) Pressure applied over the seat of injury produces... "blocked shock" or "nerve block", which means that by pressing on the nerves running from the injured part to the brain area we inhibit or prevent the transmission to the brain the knowledge of injury;

4) Pressure over any bony eminence injured, or pressure applied upon the zones corresponding to the location of the injury, will tend to relieve pain, but if the pressure is strong enough and long enough it will frequently produce an analgesia, or insensibility to pain, or even a condition of anesthesia.[1]

Later it is written, "With the relief of nerve tension—consciously or unconsciously exerted—there necessarily follows a relief in either the constricted or the congested condition of the lymphatic glands or ducts, the thyroid and other ductless glands, and also on the vasomotor nerves, which control the flow of blood through the blood vessels.

This action, no doubt, accounts for the marvelous results which zone therapy has produced in the treatment of glandular and circulatory diseases—whether due to nervous, or physical causes."[2]

Subsequently, Fitzgerald states: "We are repeatedly called upon for the theory of zone therapy. Many theories are interesting but not conclusive, and rather than be obliged to retract theories, we are not going to attempt to advance them, except very superficially, in accordance with clinical facts. It is certain that control centers in the medulla are stimulated, as had been suggested. Some theories have pointed out, perhaps rightly, that 'these functions may be carried out by the pituitary body through the multiple nerve paths from it.'

"We know that we induce a state of inhibition—a state which prevents the transmission of the nerve impulse from the brain—throughout the zone where pressure is brought to bear. We know that when inhibition or irritation is continuous, many pathological processes disappear. We are certain that lymphatic relaxation follows pressure.

"The theory advanced by Dr. Bowers: 'that inasmuch as there are admittedly ultra-microscopic bacteria, it is more than likely that in the light of this work there are ultra-microscopic connections analogous to those we call nerves.'"[3]

W. D. Chesney, M.D. reports in his work *"Zone Therapy is Scientific"* about a conference he attended—no year is given for the date January 20th, but it was probably in 1941—in which

Fitzgerald "presented charts that in his opinion proved there were ten zones in the human body—zones connected by nerves that carried the electrical impulses."[4] Exactly how these zones were delineated is not recorded. Unfortunately Dr. Chesney does not record any charts. There is no trace of why Fitzgerald uses longitudinal lines rather than horizontal lines as Head did to divide the body into zones—perhaps this was an influence from Cornelius. In the same treatise Chesney quotes Dr. George Starr White as agreeing completely with Fitzgerald.

Dr. J.S. Riley put forth no theories as to how zone therapy works, but he asks and then answers the question: "What is the meaning of zone therapy?" "It means the cutting off of pain through reflexes before it reaches the brain." Riley goes on to say the techniques of zone therapy involve: pressure, touch and manipulation; with the most important being pressure.[5]

Riley's therapist, Eunice Ingham, puts forth a different theory. In her book *Zone Therapy, Its Application to the Glands and Kindred Aliments*, when first published in 1945, Ingham states:.

"Is it not possible that by way of the autonomics, the endocrines are doubtless affected in such a way that a better synergism is brought about between the various important glands of this system. I quote below a paragraph from the recent edition of Grollman.

"It is now generally believed that the effects of stimulation of the autonomic nervous system

and elicited by the liberation at the nerve endings of epinephrine and acetycholine-like substances, which exert the sympathetic and
parasympathic effects respectively."[6]

Her view at that time agrees with the Soviet
perspective. It is interesting to note when she
reprinted *Zone Therapy* in 1951 as *Stories the
Feet Have Told*, that while most of the text
remains the same, this particular passage was
deleted.

Reflexology theory, according to The School
of Applied Kinesiology, can be regarded as a
system of proprioceptive nerve receptors, which
sends messages to all parts of the body.

Devaki Berkson in her book, *The Foot Book,
Healing the Body Through Reflexology* claims
that a Belgian chiropractor, Dr. H. Gillet, has
proven the spine and the feet do have a direct
relationship. Dr. Gillet feels "the toes correspond to the upper cervical vertebrae, the meta-
tarsals to the other cervical vertebrae, and the
tarsal-metatarsal joints to the thoracic vertebrae." Berkson goes on to say, "Dr. Lindberg, an
American chiropractor, found a direct relationship between the talus bone of the foot and its
joint with adjacent bones, to the fifth lumbar
vertebrae of the spine. Thus when one does a
plexus pull and ankle rotation...one directly
affects and releases the lower back as well as
the nerves to the genitals and lower parts of the
body."[7]

Kevin Kunz and Dr. Ralph Alan Dale explain
reflexology using the reiteration theory. They
feel reflexes in the feet are actually reflections
of different parts of the body, and the location

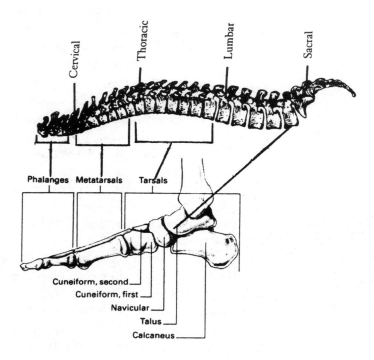

Fig. 40
Relationship of the spine to the foot according to
chiropractors Dr. Gillet of Belgium and Dr. Lindberg
of the United States

and relationship of the reflexes to each other on the feet follow an anatomical pattern which closely parallels that of the body itself. Dale classifies reflexology as a micro-reflex system adding that the reflexes are closely connected to acupuncture meridians. In 1975 Dr. Dale ran a scientific study of reflexology, or podatherapy as he terms it, validating its relationship to acupuncture meridians.[8]

Robert St. John, a British healer, has developed a prenatal therapy based on the principles of reflexology which he termed "metamorphic". He theorizes that life in the womb before birth plays an important part in our health. St. John found that the reflex zones in the spine correspond to the nine months of pregnancy. He therefore centered his work on the spine reflexes.[9]

Many other authors support the Eastern view of the body as having paths of energy (chi') and believe it is through these pathways that reflexology works. Working with electrical charged energy flows, Dr. Randolph Stone believes that the body has negative and positive poles and by stimulating reflex points in terms of these poles blockages can be released and balance restored. Stone's, "polarity therapy" recognizes adjustments and reflex points all over the body.[10]

In her article *Alternative Health Approaches*, Barbara Zeller Dobbs, R.N. reports reflexology is based on the following five hypotheses that are not yet confirmed:

"1) The energy hypothesis theory. Inside the organism, communication between organs is incessant. It is maintained through a complex system of blood circulating and energy linking the cells. This communication is happening thanks to an electromagnetic field and to vibrating exchanges between body and spirit.

"2) The lactic acid hypothesis. According to this hypothesis, lactic acid is sometimes transformed into microcrystals deposited in the hands and feet. These deposits stop or disturb the flow of life energy. Reflexology massage allows these microdeposits to be crushed and recycled, allowing the energy to circulate again.

"3) Hypothesis of the proprioceptive nervous receptors. According to some researchers, there may be a direct and unknown connection between certain parts of the feet and hands and organs in the body. Therefore, reflexing the feet or hands directly affects the different organs of the body.

"4) Hypothesis of the relaxing effect. Many physical problems have to do with persistent tension and stress. Reflexology relaxes the patient.

"5) The Psychological hypothesis. A reflexology massage is a wonderful way to provide physical contact for the sick person. It allows you to show care and concern to the dying person while decreasing pain."[11]

Bill Flocco, of Los Angeles, recently gave his views on how reflexology works. He writes, "No one knows for sure, (but here are) some theories:

1) Interference with release of over 2,000 different types of neurotransmitters between nerve endings;

2) Meridians are influenced to some degree depending on how focused one is on the acupressure reflex points;

3) Polarity—electrical charged energy flows;

4) Zones—I do not think zones exist other than as a mapping pattern that has many exceptions to the rule. They do not apply to ear, nose or other reflex micro systems;

5) Dr. Nordenstrom's energy flows through the musculature of the venous system. Jacques Hauton, professor of biochemistry in Marseille, France explains Sweden's Dr. Bjorn Nordenstrom discoveries in these words: "Bjorn Nordenstrom's (work has led him) beyond the concept of the biologically closed electrical circuit (BCEC) of the body to predict the existence of an electrical circulatory system—a system not only as complex as the circulation of the blood but also one which intervenes in all physiologic activities."[12].

6) Energy exchange from practitioner to recipient;

7) TLC (Tender Loving Care)—is worth its weight in gold;

8) Placebo—Research shows that one third of people in a study will improve as a result of just thinking something healthful and curative is being done. This concept is to be respected for the 33% of the people who get better because of it.

9) Rest—For many people this is the only time they slow down and do something for themselves. An hours rest is just the right thing for many people to give their system a chance to mend and rejuvenate.

"Reflexology probably works for all these reason and others as well. Time is past for any of us to hang our hats on the simplistic answers about how reflexology works," concludes Flocco.[13]

Devaki Berkson puts forth this theory in her book, *The Foot Book*. "Reflexology works on three levels; the physical, the mental, the spiritual. The physical by affecting organs and circulation by re-establishing, unblocking, and stimulating blood, oxygen, nutritional and energy pathways. Tension is released, nerve activity is balanced, and congestion and other deposits (a build up of acidic crystals, also known as lactic acid) are thrown off. On the mental level, the act of touching another human being is an effective therapy in itself. Last, from the spiritual aspect a healing force from the universe is called upon and used by both the client and the practitioner."[14]

According to Mildred Carter, "You will use the healing forces of Nature to revive glandular vitality... Reflex massage therapy compares with neural therapy in that instantaneous healing is not unknown in either of these two forms of treatment. This is probably because the same electrophysical processes are employed in both therapies, although in a different and simpler way in reflexology."[15]

In an interview, Sandy Cochran-Fritz, Director and owner of the Health Enrichment Center in Lapeer, Michigan prefers a more technical explanation. She explains the way reflexology works by saying, "The foot is covered with joint kinesthetic receptors. Manual manipulation of these receptors effects postural integrity. The proprioceptor mechanism (i.e. the process by which the body knows where it is in space through movement, position and weight) feeds postural information into the central nervous system. Proprioception can respond through chemical or electrical stimulation. It can happen that so much information is fed into the system that pain is blocked and/or ignored (i.e. Gate theory) which in turn produces relief of pain and allows homeostasis and relaxation to occur."

Hanne Marquardt of Germany says, "In practice, the therapist is going to work on the reflexes to the nerve roots emerging from the lumbar and sacral segments of the spine (on the feet) and will encounter acupuncture points without doing acupuncture. Similarly the periosteum of the bone will be probed without doing periosteal massage, and lypmphatic reservoirs will be massaged without your actually practising lymphatic drainage."[16]

Frances Tappan, author and authority on massage techniques, on the other hand, feels, "Other massage systems maintain that the connective tissue and the lymph system throughout the body are the vehicles for energy circuits of a nature not yet analyzed by either Eastern or Western medical science. It is the author's belief that when the explanation is found for the effects of acupuncture, the foundations for the physiological effects of reflexology and connective tissue massage will also be discovered."[17]

From England, Doreen Bayly writes, "The breaking up and dispersing of crystals which are deposited in the reflexes, interfering with blood circulation and causing congestion, is the usual theory put forward about what actually happens. There is also, I believe, an electrical impulse triggered off by pressure massage on a tender reflex and there is a subtle flow which brings that remarkable return of vitality to the patient even while receiving treatment. I believe the electrical impulse acts on the body in the same way that the stimulus of light acts on the retina of the eye. It has been proven that the action of the full spectrum of light on the retina of the eye, in which are embedded the endings of the optic nerve, produce an electrical impulse which is carried to the hypothalamus, from whence it is passed down to the pituitary gland, which passes down to the lesser glands, thereby activating all the functions of the body. It is my belief that the work upon the reflexes produces similar results."[18]

And finally one last theory from Margrete Teuwen of Glendale Reflexology Center who writes in her literature, "Reflex Zone Therapy works on the constitutional rather than on the symptomatic level. It deals with the person and not the illness. It detoxifies the body. Energy cannot flow along the sheaths of the human nervous system when there is tension in the nerves and the muscular structure through which those nerves travel. Reflexology relaxes stress and tension."

Fortunately, with the sophistication of modern conventional neurological research which began in the 1880's many of these theoretical points can now be examined and proven.

CHAPTER 6

REFLEX ACTION WITHIN THE NERVOUS SYSTEM

F irst of all, reflexology should not be confused with foot massage. Foot massage, or rubbing and kneading, is not the same as reflexology. Reflexology makes use of very precise reflex points. Most reflexologists feel a therapeutic effect is achieved by stimulation or irritation of a reflex point at a distance from the area treated. This theory is based on the fact that stimulating the skin (cutaneous) of the feet with pressure has an effect on the internal organs (visceral) and other parts of the body via a simple reflex action.

Reflex action can be one of the simplest forms of activity of the nervous system or one of the most complex. Reflexes are specific and predictable and are usually purposeful and adaptive. Reflexes are built into the nervous system and do not need the intervention of conscious thought to take effect. Some reflex actions are quite common and simple, such as the pupil of the eye reacting to light, or the jerk of the leg when the knee is tapped. For a reflex action to occur there must be 1) reception of a stimulus; 2) conduction to the central nervous system via a sensory (afferent) neuron; 3) transmission to the motor nerves via a motor (efferent) neuron which cause; 4) a response. In the above reflex actions of the pupil and leg, light and pressure are the stimuli which the sensory nerves cells perceive and relay as an impulse to the spinal cord where it is relayed to a motor nerve (muscle). This causes the pupil to contract and the quadriceps muscle at the front of the thigh to contract and jerk the leg up. These are two examples of the simple reflex arc involving only two nerves and one synapse (the point at which the nerve impulse passes from one neuron to another). Most reflex acts are more complicated. For instance the *autonomic reflex arc* has two efferent neurons with the message from one to the other in an area (ganglion) outside the central nervous system.

Other simple reflexes, like the stretch reflexes help the body maintain its balance. Every time a muscle is stretched it reacts with a reflex impulse to contract. When a person reaches, or leans forward, some muscles tighten, some loosen to hold him so that he does not fall. Even when standing erect the stretch reflexes in the muscles make minute adjustments. More complex reflexes protect the body from injury, such as blinking, sneezing, coughing and pulling your hand off a hot stove. These are called *nociceptive reflexes.*

There are several kinds of reflex actions that occur in the body. *Superficial reflexes* are the sudden movements which result when the skin is brushed or pricked. Babinski's reflex, or the movement of the toes that occurs when the sole of the foot is stroked, is an example of a superficial reflex. *Deep reflexes* depend upon mild contraction in which muscles are constantly maintained when at rest, and are obtained by tapping the tendon of the muscle. The knee-jerk reflex is a deep reflex. *Visceral reflexes* are those connected with various organs, such as the narrowing of the pupil when exposed to a bright light.

The body may also perform reflex actions to emotional stimuli. These include changes in blood pressure and respiration. A lie detector measures certain galvanic skin responses to emotional stimuli. When a patient complains of frequent physical symptoms that have no apparent physical cause the body converts a mental experience or anxiety into a reflex which results in a bodily symptom.

Another kind of reflex action works as a result of experience and is called the *conditioned reflex.* When an action is performed repeatedly the nervous system becomes familiar with the situation, and learns to react automatically. In this way a new reflex is built into the nervous system. In his classical study with dogs, Pavlov showed that the flow of saliva can become a conditioned reflex, not an automatic reaction associated with the smell of food, but to the bell which originally announced the appearance of food. In humans, walking, running, riding a bicycle or typing are all examples of activities that require large numbers of complex muscle coordinations that have become automatic through learned repeat action.

With the application of reflexology several different reflex actions occur both within the sympathetic and parasympathetic nerve pathways as well as the central nervous system. Treatment of patients and various experiments conducted by Sir Henry Head and others demonstrate the existence of the cutaneous-visceral (skin to organ) and visceral-cutaneous effect.

Although Sir James MacKenzie and Sir Henry Head worked independently and published simultaneously, their results agreed on many points. One of these points, according to Head, was that "areas of (visceral) tenderness bear a definite relation to different organs affected, but in many cases lie at a considerable distance from the organ affected."[1] MacKenzie defines the reflex process as "that vital process which is concerned in the reception of a stimulus by one organ or tissue and its conduction to another organ, which on receiving a stimulus produces the effect."[2] Head notes in one of his case histories, "firm deep pressure relieves, rather than aggravates, his (the patient's) pain."[3]

With the discovery that the whole body and limbs could be marked out into areas according to the cutaneous distribution of the pain fibers given off from the spinal segment to which it belonged, Head charted these areas of sensitivity. The excessive sensitiveness or sensibility to pain became known as "Head's zones" or "zones of hyperalgesia". While Sir Henry Head noted changes on the areas of the skin, Mackenzie looked at the changes in muscle tone and sensitivity of areas which share the same root supply with pathologically affected organs. By 1919, as neurological research progressed, Head's and MacKenzie's research was refined into a system. The area of skin that is supplied by cutaneous branches from a single spinal nerve became known as a *dermatome*.

Beyond doubt, Head and MacKenzie proved two things: 1) that there is a connection between stimulation of the skin, whether it be by pressure, stroking, manipulation, massage, electro-therapy, heat, cold, or any other means, and the internal organs. 2) Pathological conditions of organs cause reflex pathological symptoms in the skin, muscles, blood vessels and nerves. They found therapeutic agents applied to the surface tissue of the segment will influence the pathological conditions of the affected organ within the segment. Brunton's research proved the same is true. He showed how working through the surface nerve system a reflex action can be produced which is a great distance from the stimulus.

In 1909, some massage techniques were developed in Germany by A. Cornelius. Apparently unfamiliar with the work of Sir Henry Head, he reported on the clinical benefits of massage, which he attributed to reflex actions.

Later, the term 'reflex massage' was applied to his techniques.[4]

Reflexology also works within the autonomic nervous system. Long before the body's nervous system had been broken down into the sympathetic and parasympathetic nervous systems English physician Brunton wrote in 1878, "It is well known that, usually, irritation of a sensory nerve causes dilation of the vessels in the part supplied by that nerve, and contraction of the vessels in the other parts of the body."[5] A few pages later he reports, "The researches of Sanders-Ezn have shown that stimulation of certain sensory nerves, or of limited districts of the skin, will induce muscular action due to contraction of limited groups of muscles. It is probable that irritation of limited districts of the skin also induces the contraction of limited groups of involuntary muscular fibers or of limited districts of vessels."[6]

Organs receive their nerve supply from the autonomic nervous system through either the sympathetic or parasympathetic system. Affecting the nerves or vessels of either side of the body will cause changes in other areas due to the integration of the entire nervous system, or through what Sherrington termed "proprioceptive" action.

The skin consists of three layers of tissue: 1) the epidermis or surface layer; 2) the dermis or middle layer; and 3) the innermost layer called subcutaneous tissue. The dermis is composed of supporting connective tissue, blood and lymph vessels, nerves and hair follicles. Subcutaneous tissue mainly consists of connective tissue, blood vessels, and cells that store fat. The skin contains cells with many different functions. Cells which make up the skin act as a waterproof barrier for the body. The dermis and muscle layers support tissue. In addition, hairs and sweat glands aid in temperature control; fat cells insulate and store fuel; and sensory cells detect touch, temperature, pressure and pain.

The surface of the body can be divided into segmentally spaced regions which are called dermatomes. Each of these regions is supplied by a spinal or cranial nerve. The nerve fibers from bordering regions often overlap. The skin is the body's immediate link with its external environment. It acts to inform the body of changes in the environment through a network of specialized nerve sense organs. The trunks of the nerve from the skin go through to subcutaneous tissue. These nerve fibers fall into three groups: 1) free terminators which are pain receptors; 2) encapsulated nerves that record tactile sensations of heat and cold; and 3) nerves in hair follicles which also are tactile organs. In addition, as Kevin and Barbara Kunz speculate, the foot is a sensory organ. Pacinian corpuscles, which are found in the deeper part of dermis layer, especially in the hands and feet, record deep pressure of both an inner and outer nature. Proprioception is the registering of pressure from joint movement, while exteroreceptive is the registering of pressure from external sources.

The autonomic afferent system also conveys impressions of pain, stretch and pressure and other irritating stimuli by specialized nerves to the central part of the autonomic nervous system. Free and encapsulated nerves are found at work here also.

Similar to somatic afferent impulses, sensations may take part in the formation of reflex arcs by connecting directly with a cell in the lateral column of the spinal cord or by means of another neuron. Some neurons pass vertically and carry impulses to higher autonomic levels. While others may synapse round cells in the posterior gray column and give rise to fibers which eventually may carry these impulses to cortical level.

The autonomic nervous system does not work apart from the rest of the nervous system. A loud noise perceived by the exteroceptive system can speed up the beating of the heart thereby influencing the entire circulatory system. A chronic state of worry or excitement involving a voluntary part of the nervous system will often result in pathological conditions involving the autonomic part of the nervous system (tension headaches). The autonomic centers serve to modify the reaction to peripheral stimuli of somatic and autonomic origin, and establish harmonious interaction of structures under somatic and autonomic control (thermal stimuli registered by the terminal somatic nerves will cause adaptive constriction or dilation of peripheral blood vessels.)

Muscles form the deepest layer of the body's surface. Within the muscles are nerves which can alter the tension in the tissue both reflexively and voluntarily as Sherrington's work demonstrated. Both these tissues link up with the somatic as well as the autonomic nervous system producing vascular changes in both tissues. Returning to Cornelius' work, he observed various changes in the body when compression was applied to pressure points. First there was a reflexive action triggering muscle contraction. The second measurable change was a difference in blood pressure. And the third were chemical changes of warmth and moisture.[7]

In their work with three paralyzed individuals over three years in the early 1980's Barbara and Kevin Kunz confirmed the chemical changes and muscle contraction. They report perspiring or shivering by the clients in response to the application of reflexology. Responses varied between clients but, the foot receiving pressure spasmed. Exserting pressure to certain areas of the hand triggered a spasm of the toes and the foot as a whole.[8]

The close interrelation between the somatic, autonomic, and endocrine systems makes it impossible for pathological changes to take place in any one structure without causing adaptive changes in other structures. Capillary changes in skin segments within the dermatome supply of a pathologically affected organ have been investigated microscopically by Dittmat in 1943 and Rouanet in 1946.

Afferent pathways not only play an important part in the performance of voluntary movement they are equally important in the circulatory system. It is true that certain circulatory factors are influenced by the pressure applied through the practice of reflexology. The small vessels which lie near the surface of the feet are the first influenced. In turn, they start a chain reaction to the point of causing an effect in the circulatory system as a whole.

As Fitzgerald claims, in his second reason for the effectiveness of zone therapy, pressure does have an effect on the peripheral circulation and return flow of blood and lymph. Pressure applied to the proximal (where the limb attaches to the body), aspects of an injury will insure that the circulatory pathways are open enough to carry the venous flow along toward the heart. Reflexology administered to the feet can indirectly affect the limb or other part of the body that sustained the injury. However, reflexologists are advised never to work directly on an injury, but rather to work a referral area, a referral area being another area of the body that lies within the same longitudinal zone as the injury.

Physiologically there are places on the body where there are a large number of nerve cells close to the surface of the skin. These areas are found in the cheek, the back of the hand, the bottom of the feet, and the middle of the back between the shoulder blades. In addition, the number of skin capillaries is greater in the soles of the feet and the palms of the hands. The primary function of capillary circulation is to provide substances for cell metabolism and growth, and to carry away waste products. The movement of fluid and permeable substances through the capillary walls is influenced by effective pressure on the arterial and venous ends of the capillary field. The blood pressure study at the California Police Olympics has shown that reflexology, even though only applied to the feet, has a definite effect on blood pressure.

Since all tissues of the body depend on an adequate blood supply to function properly, the application of reflexology can benefit the body from a circulatory point of view. In addition, there is the chemical change mentioned above. One such chemical change deals with the sedation of pain. Dr. Arthur Guyton writes in *Textbook of Medical Physiology*, that sensory nerves in the skin can depress pain by, "(interrupting) the transmission of pain signals either from the same area of the body or even from areas sometimes located segments away. This explains why such simple maneuvers as rubbing the skin near painful areas is often very effective in relieving pain."

Experiments by Dr. Avram Goldstein of Stanford University at the Addiction Research Center has proven that neurotransmitters in the brain directly affect the transmission of pain signals and that the brain itself is capable of producing a powerful analgesic substance. The pituitary gland is a primary source of this substance called endorphins. Endorphins are five to ten times more powerful than morphine. They have been shown to inhibit the transmission of pain signals through the spinal cord and do effect the moods of the person.

Studies have revealed that pain signals travel along the nerve pathways to the dorsal horn of the spinal cord beginning a complicated reflex action. From the spinal cord the impulse is relayed to the thalamus, where the sensations of heat, cold, pain and touch are recognized. The thalamus forwards the impulse along to the cerebral cortex where the intensity and location of the pain is recognized. The brain then sends signals back through the spinal cord to release endorphins.[9] However, according to the "gate control theory" the nervous system can only respond to a limited amount of sensory information at one time. When the system becomes overloaded it short circuits, or closes a gate, reducing the amount of sensory information available for processing. The application of reflexology encourages the brain to produce more endorphins while the pressure also acts to confuse the body with too many sensations to respond to forcing the body to close "pain gates".

The pathways responsible for peripheral changes in pathological organic disturbances may also be responsible for changes in the opposite direction. Hartmann in 1928 describes changes in connective tissue within the dermatomes of the heart, causing heart symptoms and clearing up after treatment of the peripheral connective tissue.[10] It is interesting to note in conjunction with this that diseased organs lose tonus which seems to lower the threshold of sensitivity at a given pressure point. Considerable pressure is needed to alter the function of a healthy organ, yet if a problem exists only slight pressure is enough to make the client aware of the possibility of a problem. Therefore, the application of pressure through reflexology is harmless to those areas of the body that are functioning properly and aids those that are functioning below par. Regarding reflexes in the feet, tenderness vanishes when the affected organ reaches its own homeostasis.

Another way that reflexology works is through neurochemicals. Every tissue and organ in the body is controlled by a complex interaction among chemicals circulating in the blood stream and the hormones secreted by the glands. For instance the hormones secreted by the pituitary are controlled by chemical secretions and nerve impulses from the hypothalamus. Recent research has shown that nerves connect the thymus and spleen directly to the hypothalamus which affects the immune system. In essence, the brain controls the immune system just as it does with pain control and the production of endorphins. Again, the close interrelation of the entire body makes it possible for reflexology to affect the entire body in many different ways.

The question of reflexology's relationship to acupuncture, shiatsu, and acupressure is often asked. According to acupuncture the body is bisected into twelve pairs of body meridians or pathways which form the single energy system which maintains the health of the body. These meridians are pathways through which the energy of the universe circulates throughout the body organs and keeps the universe and the body in harmony. The acupuncturist believe that illness or pain occurs when the pathways become blocked, disrupting the energy flow and breaking the body's harmony. The Chinese, in acupuncture, developed the use of needles to unblock these pathways. In shiatsu, the Japanese use direct thumb and finger pressure on the acupuncture meridian points to achieve similar results. The Eastern concept of meridians corresponds frequently to the functions of the various systems of Western medicine.

Simply stated, reflexologists do work on acupuncture and acupressure points, only because in some places meridians follow nerve pathways, although in other places they do not. According to Dr. Ralph Alan Dale, Namikoshi indicates forty-four foot reflex points in his book on shiatsu, while Tung specifies twenty-five points. Mary Austin refers to thirty-three points that are not on any meridian paths.[11]

Felix Mann believes differently. He writes, "The nervous system is the transmission system used in acupuncture."[12] He also says organ meridians are not isolated nor do they function entirely independently of one another. He further states that the Indian points of the Chakras correspond to acupuncture points.

In spite of Mann's research and contentions, many authors believe that meridians lie outside the nervous system, and practitioners usually refer to an energy system and not the nervous system. Because Western science does not recognize energy systems, the effectiveness of Eastern medicines has been of no interest.

One interesting coincidence brought to light by Paul Toan, a San Francisco based reflexologists, concerns the relationship of acupuncture points to reflexology. Toan, who began studying years ago in Mainland China before the Communist take over, explains that on each of the twelve meridians there is one major point which is the most effective spot to work for the entire meridian. As it turns out, six of these points are found on the hands and six are found on the feet!

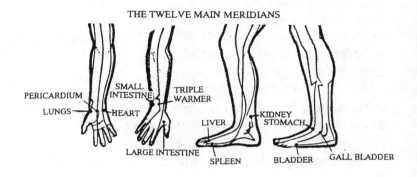

THE TWELVE MAIN MERIDIANS

PERICARDIUM
LUNGS
SMALL INTESTINE
HEART
TRIPLE WARMER
LARGE INTESTINE
SPLEEN
LIVER
KIDNEY
STOMACH
BLADDER
GALL BLADDER

Fig. 41

Briefly stated there are five main differences between acupuncture/acupressure and reflexology. 1) Those systems deal with over 400 points throughout the body. Reflexology deals with points found in the feet and hands. 2) The techniques are different. With acupressure the technique consists of applying constant pressure and holding it; with reflexology it is an alternating pressure. 3) The Eastern modalities work with points on meridians while reflexology points may or may not be found on meridians. 4) Acupuncture often works to stimulate a single organ or system into balance, while reflexology works on relaxing the body. Through relaxation the entire organism is able to reach a state of homeostasis. 5) Involves the depth of treatment. Acupuncture and acupressure usually go much deeper than reflexology does.

Without question, reflexologists will work on acupuncture points, but the theory, techniques and depth of application are not the same. In fact, a client can use both methods of therapy at the same time, as long as he allows at least two days to pass between one session and another. For when the body is given too much stimulation it may do more harm than good. Two days between treatments gives the body a chance to rest and clear out toxins.

Although it is not possible to account for all the effects of reflexology on a scientific basis, when reviewing Dr. Fitzgerald's theories of how zone therapy works, one can see that modern research agrees with his points two through four. Directly under the skin is a widespread network of nerves which receive and pass on the impulses to and from the organs. These nerves are not isolated, nor do they function entirely independently from one another although they are organized into zones or segments. Application of pressure does inhibit pain.

Even the Soviets agree with these theories. G.N. Udintsev in the forward to *Reflex Therapy* reports on a Soviet instructor in the department of physical training and medical grading, A. I. Makarova who recognizes, "the presence of reflex relationships between the cardiovascular system and the skeletal musculature, that stimulation of the ineroceptors affects muscle tone and stimulation of the propioceptors has consistent effects on the circulatory system, and that a lowering of muscle tone, in turn, has a considerable depressor influence on the vascular system, firstly, on account of reflex-humoral factors, secondly, on account of the mental influences of positive emotions, and thirdly, on account of training and the acquisition of the habit of active voluntary relaxation of the muscles."[13]

Many modern physicians are quick to discount the idea that what goes on in the mind ultimately affects the body. However, scientific evidence is rapidly accumulating in support of a "mind-body connection". Researchers working in a new field of science called psychoneuroimmunology are discovering that emotions such as love, hate, happiness or fear are linked with the nervous and immune systems. Investigators are pinpointing chemicals that travel between the mind and body proving that emotional fluctuations directly influence our state of health. This new knowledge about the mind-body connection will certainly have an impact on future medical care and its views on health.

In a recent article in the *The New England Journal of Medicine*[14] the demographics, prevalence, and patterns of the use of unconventional medicine in the United States were described. The telephone survey revealed that: 1) most people used unconventional therapies for chronic rather than life-threatening medical conditions; 2) seventy-two percent of the respondents who used unconventional therapy did not inform their medical doctor; 3) extrapolation to the population would indicate that in 1990 Americans made approximately 425 million visits to providers of unconventional therapy compared to 388 million to primary care physicians. However, it should be noted that eighty-three percent of those polled who used unconventional therapy for a serious medical condition also used conventional therapy. According to literature put out my the Office of Alternative Medicine (OAM), within the National Institutes of Health (NIH), "These findings clearly demonstrated that unconventional medicine plays a significant role in the health care system within the United States."[15]

This is one reason why the NIH has opened a new office for alternative health and is funding approximately twenty small research grants of $30,000 or less by October 1, 1993. Decisions on which studies are to be funded will be made by a peer review panel. There are seven panels. Reflexology is included under the panel for structural manipulations and energetic therapies. Examples of disciplines in this category include acupressure, chiropractic medicine, massage, rolfing, therapeutic touch, Qi Gong and reflexology. While competition for the grants will be stiff, it is hoped that some reflexologists will present proposals for the study of reflexology and help validate its effectiveness.

Currently research studies to validate reflexology are being conducted in many countries including Denmark, Switzerland, South Africa, Taiwan, Japan, and Australia. In 1990 Bill Flocco and Terrence Oleson conducted the first formal research study in the United States on reflexology and pre-menstrual syndrome (PMS). The study which included a placebo

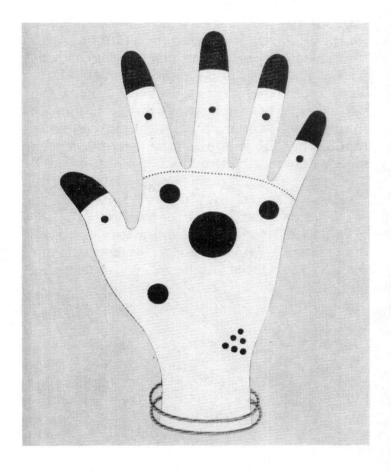

India c. 1900, zones which are regarded as cross-points of the cosmos and as chakras peculiar to the female body

routine and a special routine focusing on specific reflex areas showed a 62.6% reduction in PMS symptoms and discomfort.

Science teaches that we must see to believe. However, true science begins with an open mind which is able to observe the secrets of nature. Reflexology is not only a science but also an art. It is a science, because it is based on physiological and neurological study. Although not every aspect of reflexology can be explained in terms of traditional methods or modes of thought, that does not negate the effects achieved. Reflexology is an art, because much depends on how skillfully the practitioner applies his knowledge and the dynamics which occur between the practitioner and the client. To delve into point one of Fitzgerald's explanation of how zone therapy works requires looking at the art of reflexology. Fitzgerald refers to this effect as, "The soothing influence of animal magnetism." Whether this is animal magnetism or not will be discussed in the following chapter.

SECTION III

**The
Art of
Reflexology**

CHAPTER 7

THE ART OF REFLEXOLOGY

*C*arl Jung wrote that "healing comes only from what leads the patient beyond himself and beyond his entanglement with the ego." Dr. Fitzgerald, on the other hand, lists the "soothing influence of animal magnetism" as his first reason for the beneficial effect of zone therapy. It is not known whether Fitzgerald listed his reasons in order of importance or not, but the concept of animal magnetism is one he most certainly was exposed to in Europe.

The theory of animal magnetism was first put forth by Dr. Franz Mesmer in the late 1700's. Mesmer (1734-1815) believed that during the healing process an invisible fluid was sent out from the practitioner to the client. It was this fluid that could cure disease. Mesmer further claimed he could transfer this "magnetism" from himself to his patient without touching him. He could do this just by looking at him until the patient went into a trance. Research proved to Mesmer that when the patient came out of the trance all symptoms were gone and did not return. This technique became known as "animal magnetism" or "mesmerism". In 1784, a French commission discredited Mesmer's claim that magnetic fluids existed. The commission explained the cures accomplished by Mesmer were the results of the patient's imagination.

In spite of the commission's findings animal magnetism continued to have a following. During the mid 1800's two doctors made further contributions to mesmerism. James Braid, a British physician studied animal magnetism and called it hypnotism. Braid proved it worked, not because of some secret power, but physiologically as a response by the subject to a stimulus. At the same time a Scottish doctor, James Esdaile, found hypnotism was an effective anesthetic for surgery. He performed over two hundred successful surgeries using hypnosis.

In the late 1800's Jean Martin Charcot, a famous French physician worked with Mesmer's theory. He used it as a forerunner of modern psychotherapy. Charcot worked with patients who suffered from hysteria. Though they appeared to have physical symptoms, he showed that their problems stemmed from mental not physical causes. He found hypnosis helpful in treating many nervous conditions.

Another famous physician to use hypnosis in his work was Sigmund Freud (1856-1939). Early in his career Freud studied in Paris under Charcot. Upon his return to Vienna he began working extensively with hysterical patients. He established the theory that much behavior is controlled by unconscious motives. He later abandoned the use of hypnosis in his practice but nonetheless he did believe in its validity as a research tool.

At the same time Ivan Pavlov tried to discover a physiological basis for hypnosis. Pavlov felt hypnosis worked through the nervous system and was based on the blockage of certain nerve impulses in the brain.

Returning to Fitzgerald, the fact that he mentions "animal magnetism" indicates he believed in the effectiveness of hypnosis and in the possibility of healing occurring on a mental level. Fitzgerald must have felt zone therapy worked beyond the physical body and into other areas. This concept brings up the whole field of client-practitioner relationship, and the fact that there are many other components which aid the healing process beyond the physical techniques. These include emotional or psychological, environmental, and spiritual.

For many the most difficult aspect of reflexology is the fact that the technique is so simple, and the practitioner does not need instruments, only his hands. Actually, the best results are obtained when the reflexologists' thinking and treatment come from knowledge of human nature—whether that be intuitive or learned, coupled with compassion and love—

and not through a knowledge of disease—although a good understanding of anatomy and physiology is necessary. Holistic methods of healing, to which reflexology belongs, do not isolate a disease and treat that alone. They deal with the whole person—his body, mind and soul. The holistic practitioner does not work specifically on the problem organ or the malfunctioning system, but always on the whole person.

When healing takes place it is due to many factors. The restoration of health usually results where there occur the following conditions: 1) Homeostasis, that is the correct relationship between the body and the diseased area; 2) a balance between the body and its environment; and 3) a balance between the individual, his body, and his personal relationships—whether at work, school, home or play, with someone else or himself. Making peace of mind and spirit the primary goal is important. Rest, a change of environment, and/or a change in mental attitude will often create a healing environment and bring about better health.

In addition it has been found that healthy people are healthy because of what is going on in their minds, not so much what is going on in their bodies. They have the capacity to live life and accept illness as a teacher whatever their physical condition.

On the professional level, the relationship between the practitioner and the client has a special and important impact on the healing process. When the practitioner possesses compassion and is dedicated to his client's welfare the avenue for healing is open. Through the dynamics of the relationship between the practitioner and client a new field of activity is created, and within that field subtle forces work that facilitates the healing process.

Today the effect of thoughts and feelings upon physical health and behavior is acknowledged by psychologists. Working on a one-to-one basis, for 30-60 minutes, depending on what modalities are incorporated into a session, reflexologists will find they are reaching their clients on several levels—the physical, through touching; the mental through the release of endorphins and personal attention; the spiritual through his caring and compassion.

Given the right conditions of time, circumstances and thoughts, the healing which occurs following a reflexology session may be swift and complete. However, healing will only take place when the client becomes at peace with himself, his environment, and accepts responsibility for his own health. The primary aim of reflexology is to relax the body so that it is receptive to healing.

The problem the practitioner is usually faced with is how to help with the adjustment and release of tension at the mental-emotional level as well as the physical. Through the dialogue between practitioner and client a fresh point of view can emerge and may bring hope and relief from anxiety and stress. This in turn can bring on the change in behavior or thinking necessary for healing. To establish this relationship the client must participate in discussions which include exchanges of ideas, rather than simply receiving instructions or information from the practitioner. When the client becomes active in his own treatment by assuming his share of responsibility toward his health a positive attitude can be attained and sustained.

Encouragement can stimulate the body's defenses against disease and promote the environment in which health can be restored. Though the belief systems of the practitioner and clients interact, the client's body responds directly to his own belief. "Encouragement" does not mean lying to the client, but instead offering support and hope. Hope comes from the client's confidence and trust in the practitioner which is established through the client-practitioner bond. An atmosphere filled with humor and love will help develop the client-practitioner bond. Proper attitudes and atmosphere do not develop without effort on the part of the practitioner. When working on the client, the practitioner should try to discover what the client is thinking and feeling—what he perceives his problems to be. The reflexologist can inspire the patient's confidence by listening more than talking. Actually, if a therapist does nothing more than listen to people, the clients will feel better and they will thank you.

Unfortunately, as much as one may wish, or as hard as one may try, healing will not happen in all cases. Sometimes it is not possible to reach the other person. As Bernie Siegel says, "There are no incurable diseases, only incurable people." A client may be unable to take action. He listens, but is unable to hear and seems unable to break through or to respond to the outer stimulus. The client should be encouraged to seek other modalities or practitioners if he is not responding. For no reason should a reflexologist have his determination set on forcing the client to get better, or healing in a certain manner or to a certain level. This interferes with the client's right and will never work. Ultimately the reflexologist is not responsible for his client's health, the client is.

It is not only a good client-practitoner relationship that brings about lasting health, but some change of thinking on the client's part which enables him to make a successful conscious readjustment to his environment. Circumstances may not alter, the situation may be as difficult as it was before, but if the client has found a new way of viewing himself and his situation, then the symptoms or illness need no longer continue. Even if this does not work out into his physical environment or relationships, little by little he will find new freedom within himself and he will no longer need to be ill or unhappy. Restored health may be due to a changed mental attitude, or the discarding of, or out growing of an emotional need. Each of these will bring a slight change in the personality. With a sense of knowing options exist greater freedom or greater control of thought or feeling can occur.

There is a definite link between mind and matter. Perhaps it is this "suggestion" that Mesmer called "animal magnetism". Suggestion can be very effective yet its form is not always the same. Sometimes the quiet reassurance resulting from the feeling that something is being done to help may be enough to calm the client's fears and bring on the breakthrough to health. At other times it may be the practitioner's confidence in his ability to help that may open the healing channel. This confidence comes not from his ego but from his heart and compassion towards someone in pain. Perhaps the suggestion will instill in the client that it is possible for him to change if he gives up the need to control. The only person he has control over is himself. He cannot control how others will react to him. He must learn to like who he is or change into someone he will like. When this occurs he will control the stress he experiences from external pressures. Change is difficult, uncomfortable and often frightening. Therefore, the client needs to know that the practitioner will stand by him, without judgment, and help him through the changing times.

Thoughts and emotions are forces which affect a person's health. Of course, no responsible person will promise the impossible. However, it is a fact that the right use of positive thought directly affects the client and encourages him to hope for and expect improvement. Positive thinking on both the part of the practitioner and client, when based upon reasonable expectations is creative and stimulates a change in mental attitude which offers the opportunity for a readjustment to occur. The key is reasonable expectations. If a chronic condition has been allowed to exist for a lengthy period of time, irreversible damage may have been done to tissue. In this case a reasonable expectation may not be total healing, but a restoration of mobility, improvement in function and absence of pain due to the relaxation of stress in the tissue.

It is stated over and over by various authors on reflexology that reflexology works by getting the body to relax. Relaxation of the *mind* and body eases tension and allows the healing to occur. The practitioner is not the healer. He acts only as the mediator for the body and mind. What he is doing is to creating the opportunity, through relaxation, for the client's own powers of healing to become effective. The client, in turn, must be willing to let go of his illness in order to heal.

There are multiple factors which contribute to illness and there are multiple factors which contribute to health. Reflexology has the ability to work on many of these factors at once. It is a useful part of the healing process and can be used for psychological, physiological, mechanical and reflextive effects. Relief of pain and the restoration of function can be brought about through any one of these effects, or by a combination of them.

Above was mentioned the client's responsibility to his own health. It goes without saying that he has the responsibility to keep his appointments and be on time for them. Practitioners also have certain responsibilities. The first is to be as knowledgeable and skillful in the application of reflexology. This includes participating in continuing education and belonging to professional organizations. The best qualifications a reflexologist can have are: 1) an understanding of the interaction of body, mind and soul; 2) a positive inner attitude towards the client; 3) professional integrity; and 4) good theoretical knowledge. We have already discussed the responsibility of establishing a bond with the client based on caring and respect. Respect includes being aware within ourselves of the privilege the client gives to us when he allows us to work on him. We must always guard his privacy and confidentiality. In addition, the practitioner must eliminate any negative feelings or prejudices toward a client and develop a positive inner attitude. With some clients this will be quite challenging. Professional integrity encompasses encouraging the client to get well and giving him hope. This can be accomplished by educating the client as to what reflexology can and cannot do. Always explain what his treatment will include and what you hope will be accomplished. In order to utilize the full healing power of reflexology the client will have to free his mind from traditional thinking. He may find it strange that the practitioner uses points far removed from the area that hurts or that regardless of the problem he is experiencing, the whole foot is worked. For many people the most difficult aspect of reflexology is the fact that it is so very simple. Having a good theoretical knowledge of reflexology will give you confidence and give your client faith in your ability to help him.

Another thought to keep in mind is that reflexology is a creative art and requires the hard work, practice and devotion that all forms of creativity do. Therefore, it is important when approaching reflexology, or any healing modality, that the practitioner have an understanding of man's true nature and a belief in the healing techniques chosen for use. Studies have proven that when a doctor believes in, or is interested in, the remedy he prescribes, the results are better than when he is doubtful or indifferent. The same holds true for reflexologists. If you know and believe in what reflexology can accomplish then you will have the best results possible.

CHAPTER 8

REFLEXOLOGY BY REFLEXOLOGISTS

Thoughts, Techniques and Discoveries by Various Reflexologists

*T*here are many practitioners, with a few gems of knowledge, who do not have enough new techniques to fill a book, or have not had an opportunity to write a book. Nevertheless it is important that their insights be passed along. Therefore, several reflexologists were invited to contribute to this section. They were instructed to submit only points and techniques not found on any chart, or if located on charts, to share new meaning for old reflex points. The reflexologists who aided in this chapter make no claims that their way is the right way or the only way. They have simply found their contributions to be effective for them and their clients.

Which Foot Is Best To Start A Session With?

$\mathcal{A}$s you are aware, there are as many ways to work the foot as there are reflexologists. Amongst practitioners there is always an on-going controversy as to which foot to begin a session with. Those trained by the International Institute of Reflexology in the Ingham/Byers method are taught to begin on either foot in the diaphragm area. Once the client is relaxed the foot is then worked in a systematic way so nothing is missed, this usually means the bottom of the foot from toes to heel. This is followed by working the top and last the sides of the foot. Once completed, the second foot is worked in the same manner.

Joel Swartz of Rochester, New York begins with the right foot or the foot presented to him. For weeks, Joel says, he will start on the right foot of the client. Switching he will start on the left for awhile.

Dr. Harvey Lampell, who practices in San Francisco recommends that you start on the foot that corresponds to the side of the body with the least symptoms. In this way, by the time you work on the other foot, many of the symptoms will already be lessened. Beyond this, he says, "I personally feel that the order of working the foot should be up to the discretion of the practitioner."

"The body stores toxins, on the left, in the descending colon. One needs to release those toxins first. Then when you work on the right foot, the toxins from the right side of the body have a place to empty into," advises Loise Walstrom of Roseville, California. Sacramento's Betty Little reports that two chiropractors she knows observed in their practices that patients had no reactions of faintness or nausea when they started adjustments on the left side of the body, but did when they started on the right.

George Parnell, on the other hand, starts on the right foot and says his clients have never experienced any reactions. Argues George, "I have started on the left foot, and have had my client get sick. It seemed that the whole body system was in reverse. But, when I started on the right foot, I was following the food intake and digestive system; the toxins and waste were moving in the right direction. Take the elimi-nation system: You need to work the liver first because it produces bile. And bile helps in the release of a bowel movement. Next, by working the ascending colon then the transverse, and last, the descending colon you are working with the natural flow of that system.

"I find by starting on the right foot, working the great toe thoroughly, then the reflex area to the right lung, which is larger than the left one, gets a good flow of oxygen started. Next I work the reflexes to the shoulders, ridges, and small toes. This is followed by working the reflex to the lungs which is located on the top of the foot. Then I move on to the reflex area for the adrenal gland, and work across the foot to the liver and gall bladder reflexes. From here I go to the reflex points which correspond to the small intestines; the ileo-cecal valve; and the heel. This is followed by working the reflexes to the lymph system on the outside of the heel. The reflexes to the ovary, hip, back, sciatic, Achilles tendon on the side of the foot are next. I finish by working the reflexes found on the inside of the foot: The uterus/prostate, Fallopian tubes/groin and inside sciatic," explains Parnell.

Foot Reflexology Awareness Association (FRAA) of Southern California President, Jim Ingram also likes to start on the left foot. "I find I get better results by starting on the left foot unless there is a physical trauma on that particular side, then I would start with the right side. I consider the reflexologist as reconnecting any area of the body that is not receiving electrical impulses to a given area. I see the left side being the intake or negative side and the right side the output or positive side. For example, if you wanted to start your car you put the positive to the negative to reconnect the electrical flow, and I feel the same thing happens when you start on the left," reports Jim.

May Post, from Pennsylvania worked both feet simultaneously. She wrote, "Reflexology stimulates all glands and organs. Therefore, because many are on both sides of the body, alternating from foot to foot, stimulating EACH system TOTALLY makes good sense. This systematic flow enhances Mother Nature by working each individual body part as a unit even though half is on the left foot and the other on the right. When you think of it, there is nothing like stimulating both sides of the pituitary gland in the beginning of a foot-workout so this important gland can be fully functioning during the rest of the session, sending a FULL signal to all the glands and producing and regulating all those hormones.

"This calculated systematic approach, moving from foot to foot, system by system, enhances the organ and glandular system to do their own functions better plus work together in a balanced manner. Chronic constipation is a perfect case in point. To do the colon, start with the ileo-cecal valve, moving up and across the right foot, then across and down the left, being sure to snake across the heel then up to the anal opening. If the person tells you he or she has a problem, simply retrace the colon going backwards, but pulling the thumb down rather than the usual thumb walking action. This way impactions are loosened. If the problem persists, working the pancreas and gall bladder areas at the same time with both thumbs, then both thumbs toward the middle of the foot will get the enzymes from each organ together. These enzymes are so necessary for the colon to function properly.

"This working with the interrelationships of the organs and glands makes the person feel centered, balanced and relaxed. Imagine the body superimposed on the bottom of the feet. Starting at the top and working across and down the feet, lowering system by system, the person literally feels tension and stress melt away both inside and out. Thumb pressure varies from client to client. Tender feet are pressed lightly for the most part for a few workouts. Then heavier pressure is good around the neck, shoulders, adrenals, sciatic, and spine reflexes. But heavy pressure at first only makes the person cringe in pain, counteracting re-flexology's main purpose: relaxation," con-cluded Mrs. Post.

Mildred Carter recommends a similar ap-proach. "It is best to start a session by working the pituitary and pineal reflexes, usually on both feet. Check all toes for sore spots, includ-ing the very tips of them. Now that you have massaged all of the reflexes in the toes on the left foot, switch over to the right foot. After this you will change back to the left foot and start to massage the reflexes to the spine. After this change you will not change feet again until you have mastered every reflex in the left foot. You will find that you will get the best results this way, and you are sure to stimulate every gland and organ and nerve center of the body without missing any," she advises.

Techniques

*G*eorge Parnell offers three suggestions that he finds give him the best results. "When completing the work on the ridges, or the areas between the metetarsal bones, on the top of the foot, just before starting the toes, it is rewarding to pull the webs between the toes with the thumb and finger; this helps the lymph to start flowing. Second, when working the great toe, I have had good results in working the root of the nail. This is the reflex to the cerebellum. The cerebellum is involved in reflexes concerned with the maintenance of normal postures and equilibrium. This I believe is an especially im-portant spot to work if a client has any problems with dizziness. My third suggestion is that when reflexes are very tender they can be relaxed and helped by working the spine reflex area which corresponds to the area in the actual spine where the nerve to that organ or gland would be located," advises George.

"The technique, that I have developed concerns the rim of the heel," shares Jim Ingram. I believe the rim of the heel represents a possible block in the Achilles tendon area, back of the legs, hip area, the back and as far up as the back of the head. This is a helper area or referral area to the spine. The thumb walking technique or rolling technique is used around the rim of the heel to relieve stress in all of those parts of the body I mentioned. Working the rim of the heel on clients who have had whiplash, has many times relieved the stress in the neck area. For self-help I recommend rolling the rim of the heel on a rubber ball or a foot roller. This helps relieve soreness in the back area."

Jim also says he works one foot completely before going on to the next using the thumb walking techniques 90% of the time. "After working both feet I give extra attention to the areas that are sore or not relaxed. I do this by holding a trauma area on both the feet at the same time until I feel a pulse. Important reflexes to hold are the adrenals, and pituitary."

Jim goes on to remind reflexologists of often missed or over looked reflex areas that need to be worked. On the lateral side of the foot, where the heel meets the instep Jim finds an area which he feels corresponds to the jaw and is a good place to work for TMJ problems. He cau-

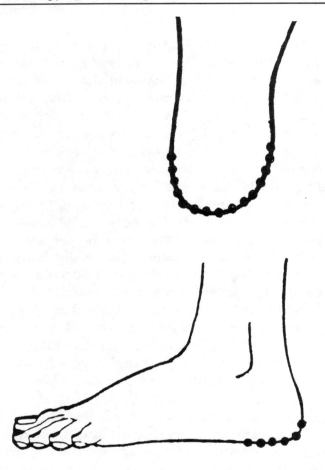

Fig. 42
New reflexes for the rim of the heel on both feet
by Jim Ingram

tions it is important not to miss working the sides of the toes and fingers. "Be sure to stimulate the ends of the fingers too. I have helped headaches, stiff necks, ear aches and stomachs problems working the area on the tip of the fingers. It seems this is a sensory part of the hand, but today with long finger nails in fashion, that sensory stimulation is gone," theorizes Ingram.

Robert Young of Baltimore, Maryland in working the thoracic spine reflex finds that the fleshy "corner" of the longitudinal medial portion of the foot reflects the erector spinae muscles, and on the metatarsal bone itself is the reflex area for the vertebrae. So he works both and often finds a difference in sensitivity levels between one foot and the other. Also, on a particularly sensitive area or point, he will tell his client to take a deep breath, while he holds the pressure constant. The client then lets him know when the sensitivity lets-up. Young believes that the more acute or recent the imbalance or trauma the area is reflecting, the more recent the onset, even if there may be no symptoms; and the corollary, the more chronic a condition, the slower the let-up.

Ulla Meyerhof was trained by Hanne Marquardt in her native Germany, and currently resides in Santa Cruz, California. Like Ingram she also believes in holding a reflex point. Ulla doesn't use much thumb walking, but instead, uses more of an acupressure technique. She locates the reflex point and applies pressure. In a recent lecture she said, "I keep pressure on a spot until I feel the response of the body in the form of a pulse. When the pulse is there I know the body is working on it and there is no reason to pursue it further. You must wait for the response of the body and trust the body will take care of the problem."

Walt Gosting, editor of FRAA's newsletter *In Step* agrees. He offers this technique for easing the discomfort found with some reflex points. "When pain is experienced in an area on the foot, it can often be 'erased' by 'fanning' or quickly stroking with the palm or back of the hand over the area."

Podiatrist Dr. Harvey Lampell writes, "Most reflexology courses recommend working the toes only to the web spaces (where seemingly the toes end). I strongly recommend when working the toes to work them from either direction, starting or ending at the metatarsal-phalangeal joints. This will ensure that the neck and shoulder muscles are handled more effectively, as well as all the other reflexes located in this area." Lampell also stresses working the spinal reflexes longitudinally. He recommends that spinal reflexes be worked from side to side. "Since muscles contract or shorten, and since most of the muscles in the foot run longitudinally the length of the foot, I recommend spending a lot of time working perpendicular to the length of the muscles, or across the width of the foot," he explains.

Dr. Lampell has a unique way of giving a treatment. He starts off with a paraffin bath. He dips the client's feet in paraffin and then covers the feet with a plastic bag. The feet are then wrapped in a towel to keep the heat in. This helps to relax all the soft tissues of the feet and improves the circulation in the feet. After 15 minutes he removes the paraffin and throws it away. He is now ready to begin working.

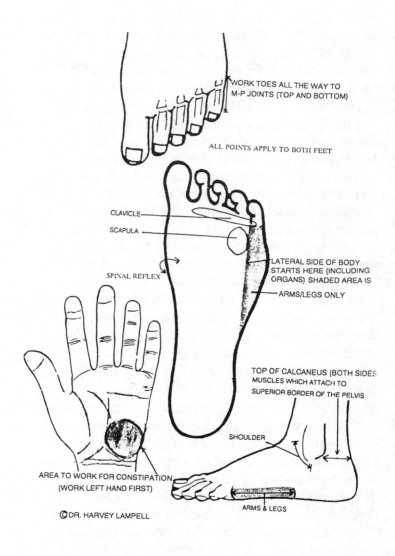

Fig. 43
New reflexes by Dr. Harvey Lampell

"I believe that bones out of place in the foot will affect the results that you can achieve. I release any soft tissue adhesions present in the foot and then, as a podiatrist, I reset any bones that I find out of place. I intersperse movement of the bones with relaxation of muscles through the application of reflexology. I have found that when you press on a joint and it's painful, that indicates a bone is out of place. Coincidentally most reflexes are located over joints. I find if the bone is slipped back in place the reflex is no longer sensitive. If a bone is out of place the whole muscle is affected, not just the area over the joint. A footsie roller, which is a special wooden roller with deep ridges carved into it, available in most health food stores is a help. When rolled under the foot it will stretch the muscles of the foot like nothing else will. I recommend one to all my patients."

"I have also found specific reflex areas for the clavicle and scapula. Furthermore, I find the lateral side of the body starts in what is generally called the fourth zone. This moves the reflexes to all the organs over toward the center of the foot. Zone five to me represents ONLY the arms and legs. In addition there is a place—at the top of the calcaneus on both sides of the foot—which corresponds to the muscles that attach to the superior border of the pelvis. I find another shoulder reflex around the ankle. Finally, the heel of the left hand is a good area to work for constipation."

Here are some tips from Mary Lou Vanderlaan of Crown Point, Indiana. Mary Lou was originally trained by Eunice Ingham twenty-five years ago. She is sold on reflexology as are nine other members of her family, including husband Bill, who practice reflexology.

"Fainting - I hit the ileocecal valve reflex first and then the pituitary second. You can't hit the ileocecal valve reflex without the person taking a deep breath. Taking this deep breath brings them right out of the faint.

"Epilepsy - On one client we located the problem as an electrical deficiency in the back of the neck. We could do a cervical lift to stop the seizure. Every time this boy in junior high played ball and used his arms for throwing it would bring on an attack. Colors would also bring on a seizure. When the boy had a seizure we would get a call from the school. Four of us reflexologists would respond, and under police escort get to the school. We would work hand and foot reflexes. With a grand mal we were able to shorten his unconscious time down to 10-15 minutes.

"If he had a half an hour on us we could still shorten the time down by 10-15 minutes. Basically we worked the pituitary on the side that was affected. We worked hands and feet on the same side. Then we'd switch and work the other side. It was difficult because he would lie in a spasm. After working on him he would sleep beautifully and wake without the after effects most people go through from taking drugs.

"Impaired hearing - I worked on a man who didn't know he had lead poisoning. He would take aspirins because of the symptoms. One of the problems he had was a loss of hearing. The sigmoid colon would bind up because of the aspirins he took to offset his symptoms. After I worked on him he could hear for a day or two. That's because the sigmoid reflex is in the same zone as the ear reflex. After he was diagnosed as having lead poisoning and that was cleared up and he stopped taking aspirins he never had another problem with his sigmoid or his hearing. With all kinds of arthritis you will find the sigmoid closed too.

"Reading marks on the body - A hardened scar on the body can develop years later into a referral pain or problem. If your client has a scar, check out the reflex point that goes to that referral area. If it's tender work out the tension.

"Blue spots on the feet - Within 10-24 hours or sooner of an automobile accident check out the feet. You will find blue spots, that aren't bruises on the feet. They will indicate where the body has been injured. These spots will look like bruises or perhaps like a spider web. After 72 hours they will disappear. It is best if you can observe the feet in the emergency room."[1]

Miscellaneous Tips

*G*oing back in history, Elizabeth Ann Riley, wife and co-worker of Dr. Joe Shelby Riley, writes about her technique for applying pressure. It is different than that used by most reflexologists today. In their correspondence course on zone therapy she says, "After determining the pain in the reflex start with a rotary movement and then press with a twisting motion and hold until the pain subsides."[2]

Richard Vise of New Hope, New Jersey told reporter Joyce Persico something interesting he discovered. Writing for a Trenton, New Jersey newspaper *The Times* Persico interviewed Vise as part of an article on reflexology. During their meeting Persico asked him how a reflexologist knows it's really the sinuses that are responding when he presses into the tops of the toes and not just an abused foot? Vise replied, "One gets intuitive, if I feel heat and constriction, it's something wrong with the foot. If there's discomfort and it's cold, it's usually the zone that's responding."[3]

Do you find yourself yawning when working on a client? Franz Wagner has this to say about that phenomena. "Yawning, coughing or sighing by the practitioner should not be suppressed, they are all signs that the body is freeing itself of disturbed energy. It is sensible to tell the patient about this, in case he misinterprets your yawning."[4]

The above suggestions regarding techniques are food for thought. Whatever techniques he uses the reflexologist needs to let his fingers tell him where the body needs to release tension and how long to work on an area.

Broadening our Horizons

*W*hen reflexologists think of their profession perhaps they should consider including themselves in the larger field of *reflexotherapy.*

Reflexotherapy as defined in the 1986 edition of the *International Dictionary of Medicine and Biology* is the: "therapeutic effect achieved by stimulation or irritation at a distance from the area treated." From one aspect this is a recognition of the neurological relationship that exists between the sensory receptors in the skin and underlying tissue, and the nervous system. It can therefore be said that reflexotherapy is based on the relationship that exists between the cutaneous and subcutaneous tissue and the internal organs, muscles, glands and structures. Considering this viewpoint, reflexology is certainly within the scope of reflexotherapy.

Like Sir Henry Head and his contemporaries, reflexologists believe that a therapeutic effect can be achieved by stimulation at a distance from the area where the problem lies; that the application of a stimulus on one part of the body can affect a different part of the body. To excite the activity of a response different stimuli or a combination of stimuli may be utilized. These can include the use of temperature (heat or cold), pressure, light and/or color, vibration and/or sound, and electricity. Any or all of these stimuli may be applied to specific reflex points or areas located on or below the skin to create a response.

For example, heat can be applied in conjunction with the use of electricity through a heating pad, or chemically with a mustard plaster or products like Ben-Gay, or with light and/or color as in the use of a heat lamp. Pressure too can be applied in different ways. It can be applied only with the hands, combined with implements, or vibration via a vibrator, or chemically with lotions, creams or oils.

Looking again at the *International Dictionary of Medicine and Biology*, the correct word for producing, increasing or predisposing a reflex action to occur is *reflexogenic*. The word reflexology on the other hand medically means, the study of the reflexes. Reflexologists do not study and work with reflexes from the conventional point of view held by the fields of physiology, neurology or psychology. Our work is really reflexogenic—that is, providing the stimulation that produces a reflex action to occur. With this is mind, can it not be more accurately said that we are not reflexologists, but instead are reflex therapists practicing reflexogenics as a specialized branch of reflexotherapy?

Generally speaking reflexologists are currently of the opinion that 1) the body is reiterated, on the feet and hands; 2) the body can be divided into a system of zones; and 3) the application of pressure to one part of a zone can have an affect on everything within that zone. These statements all appear to be true, however, let us not limit ourselves. The statement that the body is only mirrored on the hands and feet can be restricting. According to different researchers and cultures there are other areas on the human frame where the entire body is reflected. These include the ears, face, head, nose, and eyes.

Even science, itself, recognizes that each part of the body is represented by specific areas on the surface of the cortex of the brain known as the sensory homunculus and the motor homunculus. As a side note the more sensitive a particular part of the body is to stimuli, the greater is its area of the cortex. In both cases the regions needed to interpret messages from the hands and feet are two of the largest areas on the surface of the cortex.

In essence what we are talking about in either instance is the concept that the body is composed of small systems, which contain mini-maps of the entire body. These small systems are then encompassed in a larger organization, called the human body. This idea of mini-systems within a macro-system has once again a parallel in physiology. Individual cells combine to build tissue. Then groups of similar tissue make up organs and organs working together constitute a system. Finally, the different systems form a body. However, all cells contain DNA which holds the blueprint of the entire body. These systems are all connected, as Sherrington proved, through the inter-related communication of the nervous system. The entire body unconsciously responds to a stimulus which results in the occurrence of a reflex action. Cannot all these systems where the body whole is reflected in a small area be included in reflexotherapy or the practice of reflexology?

Often reflexologists view disease and treatment similar to the way conventional medicine does. That is, they view sensitive areas on the foot in isolation. When they have found an area of sensitivity, they looked at their chart, and deduced that the client must have a problem in

System	Components	Interacts primarily with these systems
Integument	Skin & Its Derivatives--sudoriferous, sebaceous, sweat and mammary glands, hair	Sensory & nervous
Skeletal	Bones, cartilage & ligaments	Muscular
Muscular	Muscles, tendons, fasciae, aponeruroses	Nervous & circulatory
Digestive	Mouth, pharynx, esophagus, stomach, small & large intestines, salivary glands, liver, gall bladder, pancreas	Urinary, endocrine, sensory
Circulatory	Heart, arteries, arterioles, veins, venules, capillaries	Lymph & respiratory
Lymphatic	Lymphoid tisue, lymph nodes, lymph capillaries, lymph vessels, right lymph duct, left thoracic duct, thymus gland, spleen, tonsils	Circulatory
Urinary	Kidneys, urinary bladder, ureters, urethra	Skin, respiratory (lungs), digestive (intestines), reproductive (in males)
Respiratory	Lungs and air passageways	Circulatory, lymph, urinary systems
Nervous	Central Nervous System (brain, spinal cord), Peripheral Nervous System (12 pairs cranial nerves, 31 pairs spinal nerves), Autonomic Nervous System (Autonomic nerve ganglia, nerves, 2 sympathetic trunks)	All systems
Sensory	Eyes, ears, nose, tongue	Integumentary & nervous
Endocrine	Pituitary, thyroid, parathyroid, adrenal, pancreas, glands, gonads---ovaries & uterus, testes & prostate	Nervous & circulatory

Chart 1

171

the corresponding organ or gland of the body represented on the chart. In addition, they often learn from symptomatical charts of diseases. As an example, for anemia, one is taught to work the spleen and liver. This results in a symptomatical orientation—the same approach conventional medicine takes. When this happens the reflexologist becomes a technician, not a therapist.

As can be seen by the accompanying chart, all systems of the body are interdependent. No one system can function on its own. Some organs or glands are components of more than one bodily system (the hypothalamus, while a bundle of nerves, sparks the pituitary into action, and is therefore a part of the endocrine system as well as the nervous system). Or components can be combined in a different way to form a new system. For example, the liver, which eliminates toxins and the intestines could be combined with the urinary system and skin and thought of as part of an elimination system.

We cannot see with our eyes (sensory system) without the aid of the brain. The brain (the nervous system) interprets the sensory signals and then instructs the muscles (muscular system) to respond, but the bones are needed to assist the muscles (skeletal system). If what we see frightens us activity in the brain sparks the hypothalamus which secrets a hormone and then sends messages to the adrenal glands (the endocrine system is now involved) to secrete stress hormones to prepare the body for action and helps produce a wide range of changes in

the body, including a near-shut down of digestion (digestive system), emptying of the bladder
(urinary system), increased blood pressure and
heart rate (circulatory/lympathic systems),
breathing quickens (respiratory system), and
the palms become sweaty (integument system).
In an instant all the systems of the body have
responded. This chain of physiological events is
often called the fight-or-flight-response.

From this example you can see that to sim-
plify reflexology by saying a certain spot corresponds to a specific organ in isolation is not
practicing responsible reflexology. Nor is it safe
terminology. Suppose the liver reflex is found
to be sensitive and the client is told that he has
a sensitive liver reflex. Then the client goes to
his doctor and says, "My reflexologist says I
have a liver problem." (Notice how the client has
changed the wording.) "Ok, I'll confirm it by
ordering a Gamma GT test," responds the very
open-minded or skeptical doctor. Then the test
comes back negative! The reflexologist has discredited himself and reflexology in the doctor's
eyes as well as in the eyes of his client—not to
mention he has placed himself in a vulnerable
legal position based on the client's misinterpre-
tation of what he said.

The solution to practicing responsible reflexology is to think in terms of systems of the
body and to explain things in the same way.
Thinking in terms of systems does not negate
the need to know and understand the function
of the different organs and glands of the body.
The more reflexologists know about anatomy
(the science and investigative study of the *struc-*

ture of organisms) and physiology (which is the study of the *functions* of the organs and parts of the body) the better. The point is that reflexologists need to think in terms of systems, not components of systems.

Through the example above reflexologists should remember three important things: 1) That a problem will often show up in the feet first. This is in advance of the organ itself presenting symptoms, or before the imbalance can be discovered with any scientific test. 2) Some other part of the digestive system can be out of sorts or stressed, causing strain on the liver. Or, 3) it could be anything which lies between the front of the body through, and including, the six layers of muscles of the back. For legal safety and credibility reflexologists need to learn the components of the systems and their function, but speak in terms of systems when talking with clients and other health professionals.

Sometimes reflexologists are at a loss to explain why it is that pressure on a certain point produces results when the reaction defies the zone concept. This is because there are other classifications than zones that the body can be divided into. Today these include acupuncture meridians, energy systems, dermatomes, and areas served by autonomic nerve function. Who knows what different organizations will be discovered and recognized by scientists in the future to explain this phenomena.

Over time, and with scientific studies, many theories will be proven. Today as we consider the information in this chapter and the next, let us not fall into the trap of narrow thinking that other professions have. Furthermore as reflexology develops professionally it is critical that reflexologists put aside their own individual prejudices, and expand their horizons by objectively considering these concepts and others which will be developed around the world and put forth in the coming years.

The Door Is Open...
Are We Ready to Walk Through?
Larry Clemmons

Larry Clemmons is a nationally certified reflexologist. He has had a private practice in the Chicago area for nearly twenty years. Larry has represented reflexology in national symposiums, videos, lecturing, teaching and writing. This article first appeared in the January 1993 issue of Sacramento Valley Reflexology Association Journal.

*T*here can be no denying the fact that every day reflexology gains more and more exposure through the media. Through television scripts, print ads and articles, the movies, or reported government investigations, reflexology is becoming a household word. As welcomed as this exposure is to most of us we must realize it is a two edged sword. Public acceptance on one hand brings more public support and financial opportunities, on the other hand it brings public scrutiny and a responsibility to provide the consumer with qualified practitioners.

Qualifications, as understood by other respected health care professionals, generally means having a standard of competency in education and practical application. The educational standard is expected to provide the practitioner with the background to intelligently converse with other health care practitioners, have a broad understanding of the anatomy and physiology of the body, and in addition to safety precautions, have a clear definition of the limits of our scope of practice.

As Billie Scott wrote in *Desert Footprints*, the newsletter for the Nevada Reflexology Organization, "As you see the push for certification and professionalism in reflexology groups, it does not mean that it will be taken away from the people who use it for their self-help and that of family and friends. However, those who are offering reflexology sessions as a business should be considered a professional and come under responsibility to the public." This responsibility includes increased education.

If we are working with the feet and hands, we should know everything there is to know about the feet and hands and how they operate. We need to know every bone, muscle tendon, nerve and function of the foot and hand. We need to know something about pathology, not to diagnose but to know when a condition is serious and warrants a referral to another professional. We need to understand the functioning of the body through anatomy and physiology.

We must also cultivate the caring side of our profession. Often time our clients will share their problems with us. We need classes in counseling to learn to be good listeners and again to know when to make a referral. Caring skills also include our ever important tactile skills. These need to be practiced in a clinical setting in an intern program like other health care professions.

If we truly desire to work with different health care personnel we must learn their language and be conversant on their level. This means we must learn medical terminology and anatomical terms. Anatomical terms are not medical terms. They are simply the common language of the health professions and are a way of identifying exactly what area of the body is under discussion. Anatomical terms avoid confusion. If I say the lateral side of the 5th metatarsal head everyone understands exactly what point I am referring to. Whereas if I say, the bone on the side of the foot, that could mean anyone of six bones on the lateral side of the foot, or anyone of seven on the medial side of the foot.

We must learn proper business techniques. Included in office practices would be learning to take a client case history. Is it responsible to say reflexology is perfectly safe and works for any problem regardless of the client's condition? If not, when wouldn't we do reflexology? How will we be able to make that professional decision, and make a referral if we don't take a case history?

The responsibility of gaining acceptance is to be shared amongst the professional practitioners, the schools, the associations, and the national testing agency.

Today, national testing offers a first step towards professionalism. This testing recognizes an individual who has met certain qualifications of knowledge and skill within the field. It distinguishes the professional from the nonprofessional. Until schools expand their curriculums, Associations have the responsibility of providing continuing education seminars leading to higher standards and training in the profession. They also can convene conferences with expert speakers and disseminate information through their newsletters. Later, schools will assume a larger role in education as their programs are enlarged to meet the quality of education outlined above. The practitioners' role is to be willing to pay the price for progress. These advances must be supported by our sacrifices of time and money. We must attend these schools, seminars and conferences. We must join and participate in associations—locally, nationally and internationally. We must do these things not only out of our love for reflexology, but because of the love and the respect we have for our clients who deserve the best we can offer.

The picture of reflexology has changed dramatically in many respects over the last five years. There are still those practicing in the home on family and friends. However, there are many others who are working professionally in private offices, in health care institutions, in health spas and in complementary health care practices with other professionals. Things have changed, reflexology had grown. A rare opportunity faces those in reflexology today as we move reflexology forward into a profession of the future. This is only possible through education, however. We must support educational programs and expand our standards if we are to walk through the open door. If we fail to walk through the door reflexology will fall back into obscurity to be swallowed up by other professions.

Whatever the outcome we will have no one to blame but ourselves. We are the future, let's do what it takes today so that tomorrow will be brighter for ourselves and for those who follow us.

CHAPTER 9

REFLEXOLOGY AROUND THE WORLD

Japan

*J*apan has several reflex systems of the feet. The first is called *sokshindo*. This system is described in books written by Shibata Watoku, however, his work has not been translated into English. A second system is *soku shinjutsu*. This system corresponds to Western reflexology more than it does to the Japanese acupressure technique called shiatsu. The words *soku shinjutsu* translates to "observation of feet and treatment of foot nerve therapy". What follows are some notes and charts I made when I studied briefly with a Japanese man. In the traditional Japanese setting nothing is written down. Students learn by observation and listening closely to the 'master' over a period of years. I am indebted to Betty Lonning of Glendale for her help in documenting this system. Located on the charts are only those reflexes that are *not* included on typical reflexology charts. The locations of organs and glands not mentioned are the same. Through the years I have found these points to be accurate. I suggest you try them for yourself and decide. If you think in terms of zone therapy or acupuncture meridians the charts will make more sense. The techniques applied are: thumb walking and pressure applied over bony surfaces with the back of the first joint on the thumb in a circular motion, and a rotary technique applied with an electric vibrator.

There are a number of significant differences with this system. The first is the belief that the body can be divided into twenty-two nerve zones, eleven zones on each foot. These zones or nerve centers are directly linked to specific body organs and muscles. A second distinction is that reflexes to the entire body can be picked up on the toes. For this reason much more emphasis is placed on working the toes.

On most clients the toes are so sensitive that they want you to move off of them quickly, but it is important to be thorough, so apply less pressure to make it tolerable for the client. Reflexes go straight through the feet and toes. If one just works all the toes, front, back and sides very well, one can reach all the reflexes in the body. For instance, a pulled muscle in the middle of the back can be picked up through the bottom of the foot, but you can actually start the release when you work the toes.

A third distinguishable idea is that any place on the foot that relates to the shape of the body where a problem exists will be a direct contact to the problem. For example, the heel is the shape of the chin and the pubic area. Any problems in either of these areas will be helped by working the heel.

A fourth concept is if you have a specific problem area, say the head, then one looks at the whole foot as representing the head, not the whole body.

A fifth difference is that reflextive therapy includes working the legs from the knees down. The knee, just above and below the knee cap, is a referral area for the neck. One can relieve neck tension by massaging that area. The lower leg, from the knee down to the ankle, on the inside, has reflexes which correspond to the spine, back muscles, colon, ureter tube, bladder and vagina. The back of the calf, running down to the big toe is a reflex to the solar plexus. On the outside of the shin bone are reflexes to the arm and leg. This area can also correspond to the upper and lower leg.

Reflexes to all glands are shown in the same place found on conventional charts except the thyroid. The thyroid reflex is shown directly down from the pituitary, while the parathyroid is located almost in the web between the great toe and the second toe.

There is also a specific shoulder blade reflex on the bottom of the foot. This reflex is usually sore on most people. One reflex for all joints in the body is located just in front of the ankle, on the top inside of the foot. Arthritics will be very sensitive here.

Work on the top of the foot to get into the stomach area. Also on top of the foot is a groin reflex. It starts between the base of the big and second toes, travels at a slight angle up the foot to the ankle.

The outside of the foot represents the head. Near the ankle you will find an ear reflex and a reflex that goes to the base of the skull. Moving down toward the little toe you will find an area that represents the head, sinus, and eyes.

As you look at the chart you will notice the entire back is found on the bottom of the feet. Remember, the foot is three dimensional. On Western charts this area corresponds to the colon and intestines. The colon and intestines sit between the abdominal muscles and the back muscles, so it would be possible to work the back from the bottom of the foot.

As you can see, the Japanese chart is much more detailed than a Western chart. But as in the conventional chart, all points apply to both feet in the usual manner. As with Western reflexology, the prime effect of soku shinjutsu is relaxation to the stressed nervous system and or affected body parts via each foot's corresponding nerve center. The stimulation of these centers provides relief to the nervous system, increases circulation and promotes the body's natural healing forces access to the ailing area. As a final note, the Japanese start a session on the left foot. This is to "honor the masters" or "ancestors".

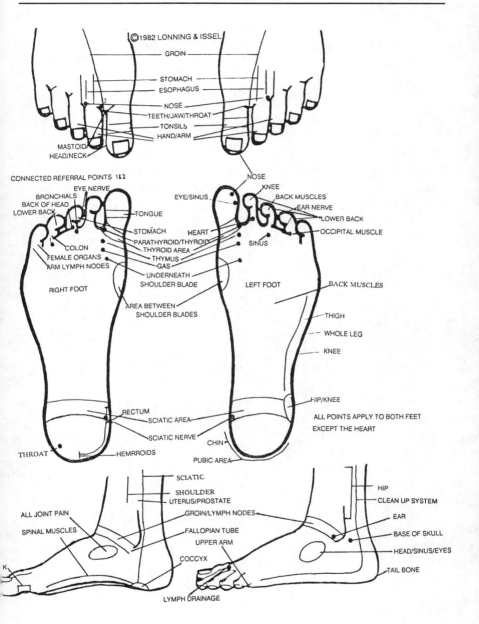

Fig. 44

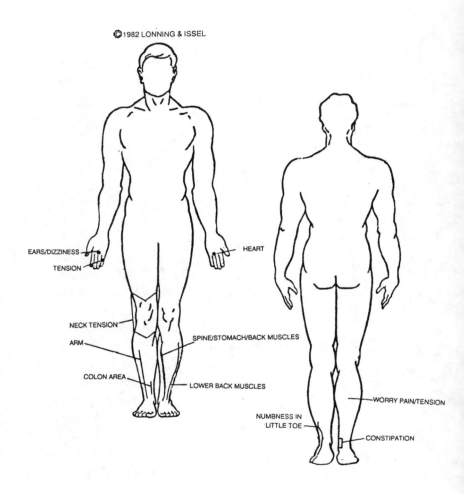

©1982 LONNING & ISSEL

EARS/DIZZINESS

TENSION

NECK TENSION

ARM

COLON AREA

HEART

SPINE/STOMACH/BACK MUSCLES

LOWER BACK MUSCLES

WORRY PAIN/TENSION

NUMBNESS IN
LITTLE TOE

CONSTIPATION

Fig. 45
Japanese Foot Therapy

Spanish Zones of Reflexes

*A*ccording to Spanish literature, the points in Fig. 39 and 40 are used to correct our physical bodies in order to give us more energy by taking out the impurities.

When working specific disorders this Spanish chart, which was translated from an Italian book, *Massaggio Zonale*, instructs the practitioner by numbers. Several examples follow. For instance, in working with *anemia* you are instructed to begin with number 34. Then back track to numbers 15-19, then work numbers 19-25, and finish by working numbers 25-31. We are told one should work especially with number 17—the pancreas.

A second example is *Angina Pectoris*. The reflexologist is told to work with numbers 21, 22, 23, 24 and then to activate numbers 15-33 and finally go down to 10.

For *breathing difficulties* numbers 14, 3, 6, and 33 should be activitated. Yet for *eyes* one works the total foot and no specific numbers are given. In dealing with *tiredness* quite a few numbers are activated. One begins with numbers 22, 23, 24, then goes back down to number 13, continues with numbers 15-19, and then 25-31. One ends with number 1. in dealing with *hemorrhoids* the sequence is 31, 52, 32, 21-24.

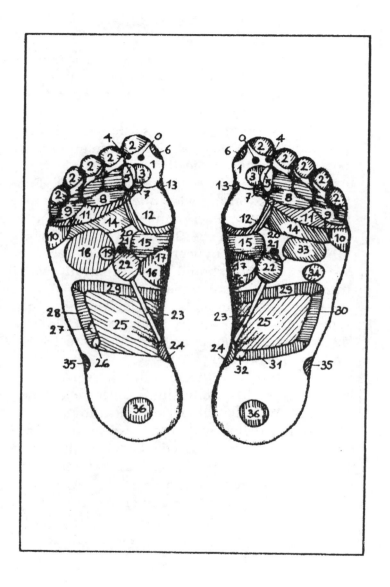

Fig. 46
Spanish Zones of Reflexes

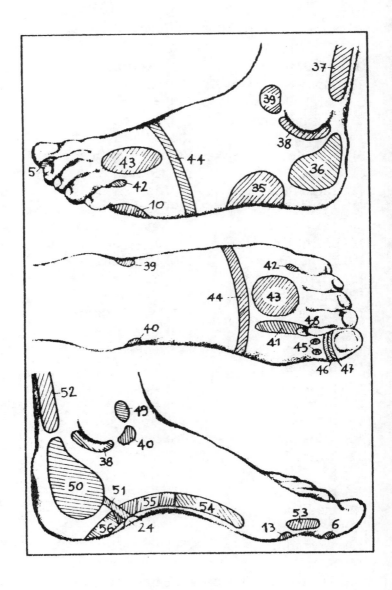

Fig. 47
Spanish Zones of Reflexes

Spanish Zones of Reflexes

(0) pituitary
(1) head in general
(2) forehead
(3) cerebral trunk
(4) pineal
(5) temple
(6) nose
(7) nape of neck
(8) eyes
(9) ears
(10) shoulder
(11) trapezius
(12) thyroid
(13) parathyroid
(14) lungs, bronchials
(15) stomach
(16) duodenum
(17) pancreas
(18) liver
(19) gall bladder
(20) solar plexus
(21) adrenals
(22) kidney
(23) ureter
(24) bladder
(25) small intestines
(26) appendix
(27) ileo-cecal valve
(28) ascending colon
(29) transverse colon
(30) descending colon
(31) rectum
(32) anus
(33) heart
(34) spleen
(35) knee
(36) ovaries/testicles
(37) lower pelvis
(38) hip
(39) lymphatic glands of the head and throat
(40) lymphatic glands of the abdomen
(41) lymph drainage
(42) internal ear
(43) chest
(44) diaphragm
(45) tonsils
(46) lower jaw
(47) upper jaw
(48) larynx
(49) anus
(50) uterus/prostate
(51) vagina/penis
(52) rectum
(53) cervical vertebras
(54) thoracic vertebras
(55) lumbar vertebras
(56) sacral and coccyx vertebras[1]

The Vacuflex System from South Africa

*T*he Vacuflex System was developed by Danish reflexologist, Inge Dougans in 1981 and subsequently introduced into South Africa. There are two steps to a session with this method. The Vacuflex System does not claim to be a replacement for traditional reflexology, but rather is to be used as a complementary method which uses modern technology. The system is also known as the "boot" treatment because it uses large felt boots.

In the first step these boots are placed around the foot and ankle. Air is then removed from the boots by a vacuum pump creating equal pressure over the foot. This applies pressure to all reflex points at the same time with equal pressure. This portion of a session lasts only five minutes. Once the boots are removed marks and discolorations can be seen on the feet which correspond to the reflexes which are out of balance and would have been found tender if pressure had been applied with the thumb in the traditional manner.

The second part of a session uses suction pads. They are placed on acupuncture meridian lines in the lower legs and arms to stimulate the body's vital energies. This portion of the session lasts about twenty minutes.[2]

Writes Dougans, "The main difference between the Vacuflex system and doing reflexology by hand is that the practitioner is only able to cover a small area at a time with his thumb, whereas with the Vacuflex system a vacuum is created around the feet which then creates a pressure onto the reflexes, thereby stimulating all the organs simultaneously. The idea originally behind the Vacuflex Reflexology System started in Denmark more than twenty years ago to aid spastic epileptic children, and it was found that hey were helped immensely. It was discovered that the solar plexus was stimulated at the same time as all the other organs, and this relaxed the spastic children and therefore their muscles could be exercised."[3]

According to a research article printed in the August 1989 issue of *Journal of Alternative & Complementary Medicine* this system was also found to be a successful help for clients who were suffering with back problems. In the study cited, eleven clients with various back complaints were tracked for 12 months. "The study showed that all types of back pain responded quickly to Vacuflex with total relief in all 11 cases after one to 10 treatments."

Metamorphic and Taiwanese Reflexology Techniques

*A*t the RRP/CNAR Fall Research Conference of 1989 two other methods of reflexology, the Metamorphic and Taiwanese techniques, were shared with the participants.

Metamorphic Reflexology
Joel Swartz

Joel Swartz demonstrated and explained the "Metamorphosis" technique also called "Prena-

tal Therapy" by Robert St. John whom he trained with at one time.

 $\mathcal{T}$ he basis of St. John's technique is founded upon reflexology. He believed that the spine reflex also corresponded to the pre-natal development period, hence the name. He calls the work as a whole "Metamorphosis" because he felt that was what was taking place within the patient—a metamorphosis of his attitudes of life.

The foundation of Metamorphosis is somewhat esoteric. St. John's work concentrated on the spine reflex only. St. John felt working the spine reflex unblocked time. It could take the client back to past lives. In working the reflex, both the client and the practitioner, were to listen to their inner being—listen intuitively to what they were experiencing. They are to allow the inner sense of knowledge to surface. The attitude of the mind of the practitioner is a large part of the way in which the response of the patient can take place.

When a practitioner is working on a patient's feet he is doing two things: 1) he is massaging and reducing the blocks and tensions in the physical structure of the patient, and therefore the blocks in Time; 2) and he is subjectively acting as a channel for energy and life to the stress patterns in the patient. Later St. John changed his view and said the practitioner was not a channel.

Although he concentrated on working the spinal reflex, no pressure is used. The practitioner makes slight circles over and over again along the spine reflex for the entire session which usually lasts an hour. The pads at the tips of the fingers are primarily used, not the thumb. According to St. John the spine reflex goes from the first joint of the big toe to around the foot at the bottom of the heel. The reflex is located higher, on the metatarsal bone, than we would normally consider the spine reflex.

Taiwanese Reflexology
Josephine Tan

Josephine expanded our horizons further by demonstrating Taiwanese reflexology. Josephine had gotten involved with Taiwanese reflexology eight years ago when she was suffering with asthma. Her asthma was so severe she was taking nine medications a day! In three months using this method she was cured and her asthma has never returned.

"In Taiwan reflexologists use a four inch long stick to apply pressure. They usually start with the bladder reflex and then work the rest of the foot. The reflexes are the same as on our charts. The Taiwan practitioner finds a tender reflex and presses very hard. If a client doesn't leave bruised the practitioner isn't doing his job! They aren't concerned with being sued for malpractice or with client comfort. Each session lasts seven minutes in total. Only the tender reflexes are worked. It hurts but it did cure me. However, later while I was in England I took Dwight Byers' course and that is the method that my husband and I practice in our Center in Singapore."[4]

The method Josephine Tan spoke about is rightfully called the Rwo Shur Method. The Rwo Shur Method of Foot Reflexology officially began in Taiwan in 1982, but had its roots with a Swiss parish priest named Father Joseph Eugster a few years before that.

Father Joseph was born and educated in Switzerland. In 1970 he went to Taiwan as a Catholic missionary. Though a young man, he suffered for years with arthritis. Conventional medical treatments did not help. A fellow priest treated him with reflexology a few times and Father Joseph completely recovered.

"That amazed me very much so that I was eager to learn this method," recalls Father Joseph.[5] He was given the Book, *Good Health for the Future* which was written by a Swiss nurse Hedi Masafret. Masafret, who had worked in a Christian mission in China wrote the book upon returning to Switzerland in 1975.

Basically self-taught Father Joseph began sharing what he knew with others. Soon he was teaching parishioners and friends. His fame spread and led to appearances on television. This exposure brought him to the attention of the authorities, and to the point that his life was threatened. At this time two brothers, Joseph and Thonet Tschen came to his rescue.

"Since my missionary work puts limits on this work of reflexology, more and more I passed it on to them," explains Father Joseph.[6] The Tschen brothers founded the Rwo Shur Institute in 1982 to propagate the work of Father

Joseph who was instrumental in returning to China the knowledge of this ancient healing method. Today the Rwo Shur method has practitioners in more than thirty countries.

"I believe our method is special because we apply much more pressure than Western methods and therefore, the results are much faster," concludes the priest.[7] Patients of this method are counselled to "be patient and bear the pain."[8]

The Rwo Shur method is named after Father Joseph. It combines ancient Chinese medical theories and techniques such as the balance of Ying and Yang, the flow of Chi and blood, and the five element theory with reflexology. There are twelve basic techniques which involve the use of the knuckles. The thumb walking technique popularized by Western reflexologists is unknown. Most of the pressure is applied with the knuckle of the index finger.

With a few exceptions, the reflex points correspond to those found on Western charts. A "balance organ" reflex has been located on the top of the foot in the hollow which forms between the fourth and fifth metatarsal heads. This reflex they feel controls the sense of balance. Another difference is the working of the diaphragm reflex. With this method it is worked across the top of the foot at the base of the metatarsal bones instead of on the bottom of the foot. The area they work for the prostate/uterus reflex is fairly large and is located on the big toe side of the heel area on the side of the foot. Just in front of this reflex is a reflex area for the penis and vagina.

The Rwo Shur practitioners are called counselors. Some of the requirements for counselors are a knowledge of "anatomy, pathology, Chinese medicine, nutrition, psychology, sociology and other clinical skills in order to enhance your effectiveness and efficiency."[9] Supplementary products are manufactured for the company so that counselors may offer them for sale to their clients for self help. These include foot massage boards, shoes, slippers and insoles, electric foot rollers, and foot ointments.

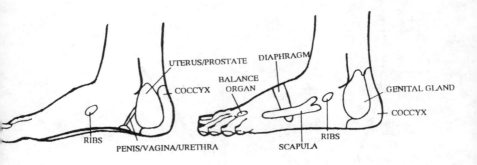

Fig. 48
New Reflexes by Rwo Shur

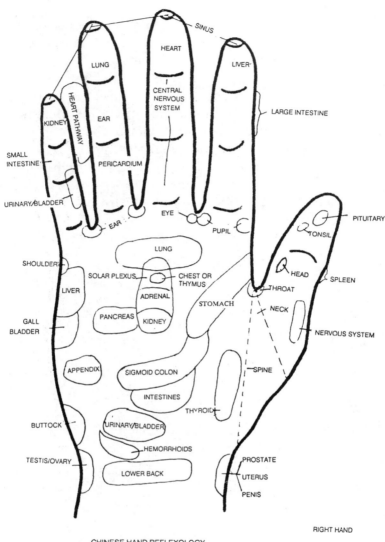

CHINESE HAND REFLEXOLOGY
ALL ORGANS TO THE BODY AND NERVE REFLEXES
SPREAD ON THE LEFT & RIGHT PALMS

© ISSEL

Fig. 49
Chinese Hand Reflexology from Taiwan

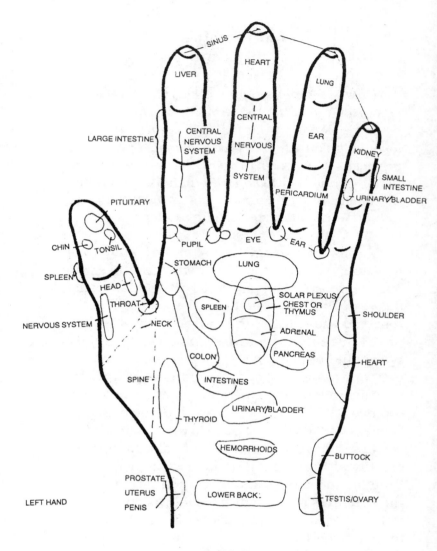

CHINESE HAND REFLEXOLOGY
ALL ORGANS TO THE BODY AND NERVE REFLEXES
SPREAD ON THE LEFT & RIGHT PALMS
©ISSEL

Fig. 50
Chinese Hand Reflexology from Taiwan

Foot Reading
Dalit Carmel

Dalit, of Israel, originally began her reflexology training with Avi Grinberg in their home country. Reading the feet is based on the philosophy below and the Five Elements of Chinese medicine. To learn to read the feet is an art which cannot be delved into with justice within the limitation of this book, but is inculded here to broaden the horizons of the reader.

$\mathcal{D}$oing reflexology isn't simply picking up a foot and working on it. The body structure not only represents the physical body but also the spirit of the body. In the soles of the feet is reflected the spirit of the individual. There is a meaning behind what we see and what we feel. We should remember a person is not just anatomy and physiology or meridians. If you want to truly understand a person you can't only rely on these. What we are is a result of the unseen. What is not seen in the body is the cause of why we are the way we are. The unseen is the emotional autobiography of the client. Everything connected, or indirectly connected, with the person is shown on the feet. It is our job as reflexologists to be sensitive to this and to learn to read what the feet are showing us.

A session goes beyond the mechanical aspect of the application of pressure. Looking at the foot we can divide it into four areas: the heel, the arch, the pad, and the toes. The pad and toes form the upper part of the foot. Correspondingly these areas can be related to the four elements of earth (heel), water (arch), fire, (pad), and air (toes). In addition to representing the element of air the toes are one place where all elements of the body are found. The 5th toe represents the element of earth. The 4th and 3rd toes represent the element of water, the 2nd toe fire and, the great toe air. The 5th element is the spine, which connects the other four elements.

We are 100% energy, just distributed differently. If there is an excess somewhere there will be a corresponding deficiency somewhere else. This disturbance will show up in a variety of ways and indicates to the practitioner how the person responds to life. Balancing this energy is vital for life and health.

Foot reading goes beyond bio-mechanics (the physical result of disturbance, which is a symptom) to the actual reason for the problem to exist. A session is an educational process. We are not doing foot reading to tell a person what is good for him, or not good for him. However, once we can properly read the feet, we can give direction in life for balancing energy simply by asking questions.

SYNOPSIS OF THE NERVOUS SYSTEM

Central Nervous System (CNS)
Function: Integrates information from PNS and sends instructions to various parts of the body.

Brain
Includes processes of reflex action, thinking, learning, memory, and intelligence.

Spinal Cord
31 pairs of nerves which branch to all organs and glands of the body.

Peripheral Nervous System (PNS)
Function: Links CNS with the body's receptors (sensory cells and sense organs), and all parts of the body such as muscles and glands that respond to nerve impulse instruction from CNS. Consists of nerves and ganglion outside the CNS spreading out from the brain and spinal cord to all parts of the body.

Autonomic Nervous System (ANS)
Function: Controls body's involuntary activities (heart beat, digestion, breathing, gland activity).

Sympathetic System
Function: Controls activities for sudden activity—increases metabolic rate (blood pressure, heart rate, glucose production by liver, dilation of the pupils).

Parasympathetic System
Function: Calms body down, often acts opposite of sympathetic system (reduces blood pressure, slows heart rate, contraction of pupils, increased activity in the stomach). Includes nerve fibers found in some cranial nerves of the brain and the sacral nerves of the lower end of the spinal cord.

Reflexology helps the body to normalize by working through both the Central Nervous System and the Peripheral Nervous System. When pressure is applied through the skin of the feet both the spinal nerves and the sympathetic nerves of the blood vessels are affected. If an organ or gland is hyperactive then reflexology also works through the parasympathetic system during the relaxation process.

GLOSSARY

Afferent - Neurons that conduct impulses toward a center, as when a sensory nerve carries a message toward the brain.

Analgesia - Absence of normal sense of pain.

Analgesic - Relieving pain.

Anesthesia - Partial or complete loss of sensation as a result of disease, injury or drugs.

Cutaneous - The skin.

"Deep" (as a term used by Henry Head) - Just below the surface.

Dermatome - An area of the skin composed of segments that are innervated by various spinal cord segments.

Efferent - Neuron that conducts impulses away from the brain or spinal cord.

Endocrine - Pertains to a gland that secretes hormones directly into the bloodstream.

Encapsulated nerves - Nerves enclosed in a sheath.

Endorphins - Chemical substances, polypeptides produced in the brain, that act as opiates and reduce or eliminate pain.

Eprictic - Acute sensibility, such as that of the skin when it discriminates between degrees of sensation caused by touch or temperature.

Exteroceptive - Organs receiving impressions from without.

Exteroceptor - A sense organ, as the eye, adapted for the reception of stimuli from outside the body.

Ganglion - A mass of nerve tissue lying outside the brain or spinal cord.

Homeostasis - State of balance or equilibrium of the internal environment of the body that is maintained by its own regulatory mechanics.

Hyperalgesia - Excessive sensitivity to pain.

Hypothalamus - A chamber in the diencephalon portion of the brain lying beneath the thalamus. It contains neurosecretions that are important in certain metabolic activities such as the regulation of water balance, sugar and fat metabolism, body temperature and the releasing and inhibiting of hormones in the body.

Interoceptor - A receptor activated by stimuli within the body.

Interoceptive - Concerned with sensations arising within the body itself, as distinguished from those arising outside the body.

Neuochemistry - Chemistry dealing with nerve tissue.

Neuron - A nerve cell which both initiates and transmits impulses.

Nociceptive - Stimuli to the brain.

Nociceptive impulses - Impulses giving rise to sensations of pain.

Nociceptive reflex - A reflex initiated by painful stimuli.

Nociceptor - A nerve for receiving and transmitting painful stimuli.

Pacinian corpuscles - Encapsulated sensory nerves found in subcutaneous tissue and many other parts of the body. These corpuscles are sensitive to deep or heavy pressure.

Parasympathetic nervous system - A part of the autonomic nervous system composed of craniosacral nerves.

Peripheral - Located away from the center.

Peripheral Nervous System - The portion of the nervous system outside the central nervous system. PNS includes 12 pairs of cranial nerves, 31 pairs of spinal nerves, all sensory nerves, the sympathetic and parasympathetic nerves.

Protopathic - Undiscriminating sensing and localizing pain stimuli.

Proprioceptive sense - The correlation of unconscious sensations from the skin and joints that allows acknowledgment and adjustments in the position of the body.

Proprioceptive impulses - Afferent impulses arising in a proprioceptor.

Proprioceptor - A receptor that responds to stimuli originating within the body itself, especially those responding to pressure, position or stretch.

Reflexogenic - Producing, increasing or predisposing a reflex action to occur.

Segmental reflex - A reflex action in which afferent impulses enter the cord in the same segment or segments from which the efferent impulses emerge.

Segmental static reactions - Postural reflexes in which movements of one extremity result in movement in an opposite extremity.

Somatic - Pertaining to the body or structures of the body wall.

Subcutaneous - Under the skin.

Sympathetic Nervous System - A large part of the autonomic nervous system. It consists of ganglia, nerves and plexuses that supply the involuntary muscles. Most of the nerves of the system are motor but some are sensory nerves.

Synapse - The point at which the nervous impulse passes from one neuron to another.

Thalamus - The largest section of the diencephalon portion of the brain. All sensory stimuli, with the exception of olfactory, are received by the thalamus. It is also the center for appreciation of primitive uncritical sensations of pain, crude touch, and temperature.

Tonus - The condition of mild steady spasm or contraction of muscular fibers causing a hard knot to be felt under the skin.

Venous - Pertaining to the veins or blood passing through them.

Visceral - Internal organs enclosed within the abdominal region—the stomach, small and large intestines, liver, gall bladder, spleen, pancreas, kidneys and ureters.

END NOTES

Chapter 1 - History of Reflexology

[1]Rivers, W.H.R. *In* - XVII Int'l Congress of Medicine: "Massage in Melanesia", 1913: 42.

[2]Kunz, Barbara and Kevin Kunz. *Reflexions*, July/August 1983: 1.

[3]Riley, Joe Shelby. *Correspondence Course in Zone Therapy Reflex Technique and Hook Work*, Mokelumne Hill CA, Health Research, 1959: 3.

[4]Ghalioungui, Paul. *Health and Healing in Ancient Egypt*, Cairo: Dar Al-Maaref, 1965: 2.

[5]elAwany, Mohamed. Interview, June 1988.

[6]Ghalioungui: 25.

[7]Watanabe, Mas. Interview, September 1990, Sacramento, California.

[8]Moorkejee, Ajit. *Tantra Asana*, Basel, Switzerland, Basilius Presse, 1971: 54.

[9] ____, *The Rwo Shur Health Method*, Trans. Geraldine Tay and Eu Hooi Khaw, Foreword by Chiao Chang Hung, Gerdine Co., 1988: 5.

[10] Hung: 5.

[11] Hung: 5.

[12] Bressler, Harry Bond. *Zone Therapy*, Mokelumne Hill CA, Health Research, 1971: 29.

[13] Kunz, Barbara and Kevin Kunz. *Reflexions*, Apr/Jun 1987: 1.

Chapter 2 - Modern European History

[1] Brunton, T. Lauter. "Reflex Action as a Cause of Disease and Mean of Cure", *Brain*, July 1878: 152.

[2] Babinski, J. *Original Descriptions of Diseases*, Univ. of Calif Medical School, Berkeley, 1928.

[3] Head, Henry. "On Distrubances of Sensation with Especial Reference To The Pain of Visceral Disease Parts I and II", *Brain*, 1883: 5.

[4] Head, Henry, W.H.R. Rivers, and James Sherren. "The Afferent Nervous System From A New Aspect", *Brain*, 1905: 99-115.

[5] Head, Rivers and Sherren: 111.

[6] Head, Henry. *Aphasia and Kindred Disorders*, New York, Hafner, 1963: 481.

[7] Kamenetz, Herman. "History of Massage", *Manipulation, Traction, and Massage*, ed. John Basmajian, Baltimore MD: Williams and Wilkins Co, 1985: 32.

[8] Cornelius, A. *Druckpunkte*, Berlin, 1902: 2.

[9] Cornelius: 2.

[10] Cornelius: 10.

[11] Cornelius: 10.

[12]Cornelius: 4.

[13]Cornelius: 12.

[14]Cornelius: 19.

[15]Kamenetz: 33.

[16]Ebner, Maria. *Connective Tissue Massage*, Edinburgh, E & S Livingstone Ltd., 1962: 164.

[17]Marquardt, Hanne. *Reflex Zone Therapy of the Feet*, New York, Thorsons Publishers, 1983: 10.

[18]Boring, Edwin. *A History of Experimental Psychology*, New Jersey, Prentice-Hall, 1950: 635.

[19]Bekhterev, Vladimir. *General Principles of Human Reflexology*, New York, International Publishers, 1932: 33.

[20]Gris, Henry and William Dick. *The New Soviet Psychic Discoveries*, New Jersey, Prentice-Hall, 1978: 272.

[21]Udinstev, G.N. *Reflex Therapy, Part I*, New York, Consultants Bureau Enterprise, Inc., 1962: 5.

Chapter 3 - The Americans and Reflexology

[1]Wagner, Franz. *Reflex Zone Massage*, Wellingborough, Thornsons Publishers, 1987: 25.

[2]Wallace, Jenny. Interview, May 1989.

[3]Fitzgerald, William H. and Edwin F. Bowers. *Zone Therapy*, Mokelumne Hill CA, Health Research, 1917: 9.

[4]Bressler, Harry Bond. *Zone Therapy*, Mokelumne Hill CA, Health Research, 1971: 20.

[5]Chesney, W.D. *Zone Therapy is Scientific*, Mokelumne Hill CA, Health Research, 1969: 3.

[6]Fitzgerald and Bowers: 172.

[7]Bowers, Edwin. "To Stop That Toothache, Squeeze Your Toe!", *Everybody's Magazine*, Sept. 15, 1915: 285-291.

[8]Dale, Ralph Alan. *The Micro-Acupuncture Systems Book II*, Dialectic Press, 1984: 4.

[9]Bowers: 285-291.

[10]White, George Starr. "Lecture Course to Physicians, Part Six", *Zone Therapy*, Mokelumne Hill CA, Health Research: 872.

[11]Lust, Benedict. *Zone Therapy*, New York, Lust Publication, 1980: 20.

[12]White: 873.

[13]Riley, Joe Shelby. *Correspondence Course in Zoone Therapy and Hook Work*, Mokelumne Hill CA, Health Research, 1959: 3.

[14]Chesney: 8 (Quote by publisher, not Chesney).

[15]Chesney: 8 (Quote by publisher, not Chesney).

[16]Byers, Dwight. Interview, Jan. 1988.

[17]Byers, Interview.

[18]Private letter from Joe S. Riley to Eunice Ingham, Sept. 14, 1938.

[19]Byers, Interview.

[20]_____, *Hospital Corps Quarterly*, U.S. Navy, Nov. 1944: 201-202.

[21]Benjamin, Patricia. "Eunice D. Ingham and the Development of Foot Reflexology in the United States", *Massage Therapy Journal*, Spring 1989: 42.

[22]Newspaper clipping in the Ingham files.

[23]Mazzarelli, Anna. Interview, Jan. 1988.

[24]Clark, Ralph. "Footwork To Cure All Ills Charged in Woman's Trial", *Valley Times Today*, Jan. 8, 1961.

[25]Goldberg, Robert. "Mildred Carter, Pioneer in Reflexology", *Whole Life Monthly*, May 1967: 50-51.

Chapter 4 - Reflexology Today

[1]Swift, E.M. "Carol and Her Big Lug", *Sports Illustrated*, Feb 9, 1987: 88-94.

[2]Private letter from Ted Cooke to Jerry Budenz, June 28, 1988.

[3]_____, "Police Olympics in Reflexology Study", *Massage Magazine*, Feb/Mar 1988: 16.

[4]Dobbs, Barbara Zeller. "Alternative Health Approaches", *Nursing Mirror*, Feb. 27, 1985: 41-42.

[5]Clemmons, Larry. "Reflexology...Standing On It's Feet", *The Massage Journal*, April 1985: 38-39.

[6]Fuller, Chris. "Unusual Ways to Beat Arthritis Pain", *National Enquirer*, August 8, 1988: 44.

[7]Cote, Michael. "Reflexology", *Rocky Mountain News*, Denver CO, Nov. 10, 1988.

[8]Schleper, Anne. "Reflexologists Says Steps to Good Health Begin With the Sole", *Evansville Courier*, Evansville IN, Aug. 21, 1988: 11.

[9]Norman, Laura and Thomas Cowan. *Feet First*, New York, Fireside, 1988: 11.

[10]Kunz, Barbara and Kevin Kunz. Reflexology Research Project, brochure.

[11]Kunz, Television and Reflexology, press release.

[12]*Sacramento Valley Reflexology Association Journal*, "Reflexology in the Philippines", June 1988: 1.

[13]Conference of North American Reflexologists (CNAR), Record of Proceedings, May 27-28, 1989: 4.

[14]California Conference of Reflexologists (CCR), Conference brochure, March 4-5, 1989: 26.

[15]CCR, Record of Proceedings: 12.

[16]CNAR, Record of Proceedings: 3.

[17]CNAR, Record of Proceedings: 11.

[18]CNAR, Record of Proceedings: 17.

[19]Kunz, Barbara and Kevin Kunz. "The Trial of a Reflexologist", *Reflexions*, Nov/Dec 1982: 1.

[20]Letter from Linda Mc Cready of the State of California, Dept. of Consumer Affairs, to John Myers, Dec. 13, 1983.

[21]CNAR, Record of Proceedings: 24.

[22]RAC/CNAR Conference Brochure, Record of Proceedings, September 29-30 1990: 36-47.

[23]Farhi, Paul. "Catch a Trend", *Sacramento Bee*, Sacramento, CA, October 12, 1990: Scene 1.

Chapter 5 - How and Why Reflexology Works

[1]Fitzgerald, William F. and Edwin Bowers. *Zone Therapy*, Mokelumne Hill CA, Health Research, 1917: 15.

[2]Fitzgerald: 140.

[3]Fitzgerald: 181.

[4]Chesney, W.D. *Zone Therapy is Scientific*, Mokelumne Hill CA, Health Research, 1969: 4.

[5]Riley, Joe Shelby. *Correspondence Course in Zone Theapy Reflex Technique and Hook Work*, Mokelumne Hill CA, Health Research, 1969: Lesson 13, 1.

[6]Ingham, Eunice. *Zone Therapy*, Rochester NY, Ingham Publishing, 1945: 29.

[7]Berkson, Devaki. *The Foot Book*, New York, Barnes and Noble Books, 1977: 14.

[8]Dale, Ralph Alan. *The Micro-Acpuncture Systems Book I*, Dialectic Press: 15.

[9]Wagner, Franz. *Reflex Zone Massage*, Wellingborough, Thorsons Publishing Grouip, 1987: 30.

[10]Berkson: 12.

[11]Dobbs, Barbara Zeller. "Alternative Health Approaches", *Nursing Mirror*, Feb 27, 1985: 41-42.

[12]Nordenstrom, Bjorn E. *Biologically Closed Electric Circuits*, Stockholm, Nordic Medical Publications, 1983: VII.

[13]California Conference of Reflexologists (CCR), conference brochure, March 4-5, 1989: 35.

[14]Berkson: 12.

[15]Carter, Mildred. *Helping Yourself with Foot Reflexology*, New Jersey, Prentice-Hall, 1969: 29.

[16]Marquardt, Hanne. *Reflex Zone Therapy*, New York, Thorsons Publishers, 1983: 27.

[17]Tappan, Frances. *Healing Massage Techniqiues*, Virginia, Reston Publishing Co., 1980: 180.

[19]Bayly, Doreen. *Reflexology Today*, New York, Thorsons Publishers, 1986: 13.

Chapter 6 - Reflex Action Within the Nervous System

[1]Head, Henry. "On Distrubances of Sensation With Especial Reference to the Pain of Visceral Disease", *Brain*, 1893: 56.

[2]MacKenzie, James. *Angina Pectoris*, London, Henry Frowde and Hodder and Stoughton, 1923: 47.

[3]Head: 71.

[4]Kamenetz, Herman. "History of Massage", *Manipulation, Traction and Massage*, ed. John Basmajian, Baltimore, Williams and Wilkins Co., 1985: 32.

[5]Brunton, T. Lauter. "Reflex Action as a Cause of Disease and Means of Cure", *Brain*, July 1878: 147.

[6]Brunton: 149.

[7]Cornelius, A. *Druckpunkte*, Berlin, 1902: 2.

[8]Kunz, Barbara and Kevin Kunz. "The Paralysis Report", Jan-Mar 1987: 2.

[9]Goldstein, Avram. "Opioid Peptides (Endorphis) in Pituitary and Brain", *Science*, Sept. 17, 1976: 1081-1086.

[10]Ebner, Maria. *Connective Tissue Massage*, Edinburgh, E & S Livingstone, Ltd., 1962: 52.

[11]Dale, Ralph Alan. *The Micro-Acupuncture Systems Book I* Dialectic Press: 12.

[12]Mann, Felix. *Acupuncture The Ancient Chinese Art of Healing and How It Works Scientifically*, New York, First Vintage Books, 1973: 5.

[13]Udintsev, G.N. *Reflex Therapy Part I*, New York, Consultants Bureau Enterprises, Inc., 1962: 5.

[14]Eisnenberg, David, M.D., et al, "Unconventional Medicine in the United States," The New England Journal of Medicine, 328:246-252, January 28, 1993.
[15]_____, NIH Guide, "Exploratory Grants for Alternative Medicine" Volume 22, Number 12, March 26, 1993.

Chapter 8 - Reflexology by Reflexologists

[1]RRP & CNAR Fall Conference Brochure, October 15-16, 1989: 5.
[2]Riley, Elizabeth Ann. "Class Lessons in Zone Therapy, Reflex Technique and Hook Work", *Correspondence Course in Zone Therapy, Reflex Technique and Hook Work*, Mokelumne Hill CA Health Research, 1959: 1.
[3]Persico, Joyce. "Reflexology", *The Times*, Trenton NJ, Sep. 4, 1986: B-1.
[4]Wagner, Franz. *Reflex Zone Massage*, Wellingborough, Thorsons Publishing Group, 1987: 56.

Chapter 9 - Reflexology Around the World

[1]Erede, Clara Bianca. *Masaje Zonal En Los Pies*, Barcelona, EMERGE, 1982: 54.
[2]Hall, Nicola M. *Reflexology—A Better Way to Health*, Pan Books, 1988: 175.
[3]Private letter from Inge Dougans to Christine Issel, Oct. 15, 1990.
[4]RRP/CNAR Fall Conference Brochure, Oct 15-16, 1989: 14-15.
[5]Eugster, Father Joseph, Interview, Jul 1990, Tokyo.

[6]Eugster, Interview.

[7]Eugster, Interview.

[8]Eugster, Interview.

[9] ____, *The Rwo Shur Health Method*, Trans. Geraldine Tay and Eu Hooi Khaw, Gerdine Co., 1988: 121.

BIBLIOGRAPHY

Babinski, J. *Original Descriptions of Diseases*, Univ. of Calif Medical School, Berkeley, 1928.

Bayly, Doreen. *Reflexology Today*, Thorsons Publishers, New York, 1986.

Bekhterev, Vladimir. *General Principles of Human Reflexology*, New York, International Publishers, 1932.

Benjamin, Patricia. "Eunice D. Ingham and the Development of Foot Reflexology in the United States", *Massage Therapy Journal*, Spring 1989.

Berkson, Devaki. *The Foot Book*, New York, Barnes and Noble Books, 1977.

Boring, Edwin. *A History of Experimental Psychology*, New Jersey, Prentice-Hall, 1950.

Bosiger, Carol. "Vacuflex Reflexology Study Shows the System Is Successful in Clearing Back Pain", *Journal of Alternative and Complementary Medicine*, Aug. 1989.

Bowers, Edwin. "To Stop That Toothache, Squeeze Your Toe!", *Everybody's Magazine*, Sept. 15, 1915.

Bressler, Harry Bond. *Zone Therapy*, Mokelumne Hill CA, Health Research, 1971.

Brunton, T. Lauter. "Reflex Action as a Cause of Disease and Mean of Cure", *Brain*, July 1878.

Byers, Dwight. Interview, January 1988, Los Angeles CA.

California Conference of Reflexologists, Conference brochure, March 4-5, 1989, Los Angeles, CA.

Carter, Mildred. *Helping Yourself with Foot Reflexology*, New Jersey, Prentice-Hall, 1969.

Chesney, W.D. *Zone Therapy is Scientific*, Mokelumne Hill CA, Health Research, 1969.

Clark, Ralph. "Footwork To Cure All Ills Charged in Woman's Trial", *Valley Times Today*, Jan. 8, 1961.

Clemmons, Larry. "Reflexology...Standing On It's Feet", *The Massage Journal*, April 1985.

Conference of North American Reflexologists (CNAR), Record of Proceedings, May 27-28, 1989, Denver CO.

Cooke, Ted. Private letter to Jerry Budenz, June 28, 1988, Culver City CA.

Cornelius, A. *Druckpunkte*, Berlin, 1902.

Cote, Michael. "Reflexology", *Rocky Mountain News*, Denver CO, Nov. 10, 1988.

Dale, Ralph Alan. *The Micro-Acupuncture Systems Book I* Dialectic Press.

Dale, Ralph Alan. *The Micro-Acupuncture Systems Book II*, Dialectic Press, 1984.

Dobbs, Barbara Zeller. "Alternative Health Approaches", *Nursing Mirror*, Feb 27, 1985.

Dougans, Inge. Private letter to Christine Issel, Oct 15, 1990.

Ebner, Maria. *Connective Tissue Massage*, Edinburgh, E & S Livingstone Ltd., 1962.

elAwany, Mohamed. Interview, June 1988, Los Angeles CA.

Eisnenberg, David, M.D., et al, "Unconventional Medicine in the United States," The New England Journal of Medicine, 328:246-252, January 28, 1993.

Erede, Clara Bianca. *Masaje Zonal En Los Pies*, Barcelona, EMERGE, 1982.

Eugster, Joseph Fr. Interview, Jul. 1990. Tokyo, Japan.

Farhi, Paul. "Catch a Trend", *Sacramento Bee*, Sacramento CA Oct. 12, 1990.

Fitzgerald, William H. and Edwin F. Bowers. *Zone Therapy*, Mokelumne Hill CA, Health Research, 1917.

Fuller, Chris. "Unusual Ways to Beat Arthritis Pain", *National Enquirer*, August 8, 1988.

Ghalioungui, Paul. *Health and Healing in Ancient Egypt*, Cairo: Dar Al-Maaref, 1965.

Goldberg, Robert. "Mildred Carter, Pioneer in Reflexology", *Whole Life Monthly*, May 1967.

Goldstein, Avram. "Opioid Peptides (Endorphis) in Pituitary and Brain", *Science*, Sept. 17, 1976.

Gris, Henry and William Dick. *The New Soviet Psychic Discoveries*, New Jersey, Prentice-Hall, 1978.

Hall, Nicola M. *Reflexology - A Better Way To Health*, Pan Books, 1988.

Head, Henry. *Aphasia and Kindred Disorders*, New York, Hafner, 1963.

Head, Henry. "On Distrubances of Sensation with Especial Reference To The Pain of Visceral Disease Parts I and II", *Brain*, 1883.

Head, Henry, W.H.R. Rivers, and James Sherren. "The Afferent Nervous System From A New Aspect", *Brain*, 1905.

Hospital Corps Quarterly, U.S. Navy, Nov. 1944.

Ingham, Eunice. *Zone Therapy*, Rochester NY, Ingham Publishing, 1945.

Ingham files, Newspaper clipping.

International Dictionary of Medicine and Biology, Vol III, ed. Sidney I. Landau, New York: John Wiley & Sons, Inc., 1986.

Kamenetz, Herman. "History of Massage", *Manipulation, Traction, and Massage*, ed. John Basmajian, Baltimore MD: Williams and Wilkins Co, 1985.

Kunz, Barbara and Kevin Kunz, flyer.

Kunz, Barbara and Kevin. Television and Reflexology, press release.

Kunz, Barbara and Kevin Kunz. *Reflexions*, Nov/Dec 1982, "The Trial of a Reflexologist".

Kunz, Barbara and Kevin Kunz. *Reflexions*, Jul/Aug 1983.

Kunz, Barbara and Kevin Kunz. *Reflexions*, Apr/Jun 1987.

Kunz, Barbara and Kevin Kunz. *Reflexions*, Jan/Mar 1987, "The Paralysis Report",

Kunz, Barbara and Kevin Kunz. Reflexology Research Project, brochure.

Lust, Benedict. *Zone Therapy*, New York, Lust Publication, 1980.

MacKenzie, James. *Angina Pectoris*, London, Henry Frowde and Hodder and Stoughton, 1923.

Mann, Felix. *Acupuncture The Ancient Chinese Art of Healing and How It Works Scientifically*, New York, First Vintage Books, 1973.

Marquardt, Hanne. *Reflex Zone Therapy of the Feet*, New York, Thorsons Publishers, 1983.

Mazzarelli, Anna. Interview, Jan. 1988, Los Angeles CA.

Mc Cready, Linda, of the State of California, Dept. of Consumer Affairs. Private letter to John Myers, Dec. 13, 1983.

Miller, Johnathan. *The Body In Question*, New York, Random House, 1978.

Mookerjee, Ajit. *Tantra Asana*, Basel, Switzerland, Basilius Presse, 1971.

NIH Guide, "Exploratory Grants for Alternative Medicine" Volume 22, Number 12, March 26, 1993.

Nordenstrom, Bjorn E. *Biologically Closed Electric Circuits*, Stockholm, Nordic Medical Publications, 1983.

Norman, Laura and Thomas Cowan. *Feet First*, New York, Fireside, 1988.

"Police Olympics in Reflexology Study", *Massage Magazine*, Feb/Mar 1988.

Persico, Joyce. "Reflexology", *The Times*, Trenton NJ, Sep. 4, 1986.

Purce, Jill. *The Mystic Spiral*, New York, Thames and Hudson, Inc., 1980.

Riley, Elizabeth Ann. "Class Lessons in Zone Therapy, Reflex Technique and Hook Work", *Correspondence Course in Zone Therapy, Re-*

flex Technique and Hook Work, Mokelumne Hill CA, Health Research, 1959.

Riley, Joe Shelby. *Correspondence Course in Zone Therapy Reflex Technique and Hook Work*, Mokelumne Hill CA, Health Research, 1959.

Riley, Joe Shelby. *Zone Reflex*, Mokelumne Hill CA, Health Research, 1942.

Riley, Joe Shelby. Private letter to Eunice Ingham, Sept. 14, 1938, Washington DC.

Rivers, W.H.R. *In* - XVII Int'l Congress of Medicine: "Massage in Melanesia", 1913.

RRP & CNAR Fall Conference Brochure, October 15-16, 1989, Piqua OH.

The Rwo Shur Health Method, Trans. Geraldine Tay and Eu Hooi Khaw, Gerdine Co., 1988.

Sacramento Valley Reflexology Association Journal, "Reflexology in the Philippines", June 1988.

Schleper, Anne. "Reflexologists Says Steps to Good Health Begin With the Sole", *Evansville Courier*, Evansville IN, Aug. 21, 1988.

Swift, E.M. "Carol and Her Big Lug", *Sports Illustrated*, Feb 9, 1987.

Tappan, Frances. *Healing Massage Techniqiues*, Virginia, Reston Publishing Co., 1980.

Time-Life Books. *The World's Great Religions*, ed. Sam Wells, New York, Time Inc., 1957.

Udinstev, G.N. *Reflex Therapy, Part I*, New York, Consultants Bureau Enterprise, Inc., 1962.

Wagner, Franz. *Reflex Zone Massage*, Wellingborough, Thorsons Publishing Group, 1987.

Wallace, Jenny. Interview, May 1989, Sacramento CA.

Watanabe, Mas. Interview, Sacramento, Sept. 1990, Sacramento CA.

White, George Starr. "Lecture Course to Physicians, Part Six", *Zone Therapy*, Mokelumne Hill CA, Health Research.

INDEX

𝒜

ℬ

F

G

H

I

J

K

L

M

N

efferent 120
Nogier, Paul 65

$\mathcal{P}$

Pain, Gate theory 130
Pain management 86
Parnell, George 155, 158
Pavlov, Ivan 40, 143
Playboy 88
Polarity 113
Post, May 156
Propioceptors 135
Proprioception 125
Proprioceptive 111, 124
Proproceptive 32

$\mathcal{R}$

Reflex arc
    simple 120
Reflexes
    Babinski, M.J. 121
    conditioned 121
    Deep 121
    nociceptive 121
    Superficial 121
    Visceral 121
Reflexogenic 169
Reflexology
    Metamorphic 192
    Spanish 187
    Taiwanese 194
    term 42, 73
Reflexology Research Project 85
Reflexology Theory

S

Z

Zone therapy 73

Zones
    Head 29
    hyperalgesia 29, 123
    Head's 54, 123

Worldwide Timeline of Reflexology

c. 2,500 B. C. Egypt: pictograph discovered by American Ed Case in 1979.

c. 2,500 B.C. China: Acupuncture.

c. 500 B.C. Japan: Acupuncture migrates to Japan.

1582 - Europe: Book on zone therapy published by Drs. Adamus and A'tatis.

1583 - Germany: Book on zone therapy published in Leipzig by Dr. Ball.

c. 1750 - Hindu paintings of hands and feet.

1771 - Germany: word "reflex" first used by Johann Unzer.

1833 - England: term "reflex action" coined by Marshall Hall.

1878 - England: Article, "Reflex Action as a Cause of Disease and Means of Cure" published by T. Lauder Brunton.

1880 - Europe: Accupuncture finds its way to Europe.

1893 - France: Babinski's reflex discovered.

1893 - England: Sir Henry Head's research published proving direct relationship between pressure applied to skin and internal organs. "Head's Zones" charted. Later refined into dermatomes.

1899 - Germany: Benedikts published: *Treatment and Healing of Nervous Suffering and Nervous Pain by Hand Manipulation.*

1902 - Germany: Cornelius publishes: *Pressure Points, Their Origin and Significance.*

1902 - Vienna: Fitzgerald studying and teaching.

1904 - Russia: Pavlov receives Nobel Prize for proving direct relationship between stimulus to a response - reflex action.

1906 - England: Sir Charles Sherrington publishes, *The Integrative Action of the Nervous System.* Proves whole nervous system adjusts to stimulus - terms this proprioception

1907 - Russia: Term "reflexology" coined by Bekhterev.

1911 - Germany: Barczewski terms "reflexmassage". Term applied to different systems which applied pressure as a method of healing.

1913 - Japan: Dr. Kutakichi Hirata charts body as translated by Dr. Ralph Alan Dale of the U.S.

1915 - U.S.: Bowers article published, "To Stop That Toothache, Squeeze Your Toe".

1917 - U.S.: Bowers and Fitzgerald publish *Zone Therapy*.

c. 1918 - England: Edgar Adrian proved the electrical intensity of the nerve impulse depends on the size of the nerve rather than upon the strength of the stimulus.

1919 - U.S.: Joe Shelby Riley publishes, *Zone Theapy Simplied*, his first of many books on zone therapy.

1929 - Germany: Elisabeth Dicke - based on concept of reflex zone massage applied massage techniques to the connective tissue within the segemental zones established by Head.

1932 - Russia: Bekhterev's work Objective Psychology which was originally published in 1907, revised as *General Principles of Human Reflexology* and translated into English.

1935 - Switzerland: Dr. E.R. Schwank spreads knowledge of acupressure throughout Europe.

1938 - U.S.: Ingham publishes, *Stories the Feet Can Tell*, begins 40 year lecturing career.

1945 - U. S.: Ingham publishes, *Zone Therapy and Gland Reflexes*. Revised in 1951 and published as *Stories the Feet Have Told*.

1955 - Germany: W. Kohlraush publishes *Reflexzonenmassage in Muskulatur and Bindegewebe*. Distrubances of the organs follow vascular channels which are associated with the reflexes of the arteries.

1955 - U.S.: State of Nebraska refers to reflexology as quackery and outlaws its practice.

1956 - U.S.: South Dakota also.

1961 - U.S.: Mazzarelli vs. the California State Board of Medical Examiners.

1968 - U.S.: State of New York vs. Eunice Ingham - charges dropped.

1969 - U.S.: Mildred Carter publishes *Helping Yourself with Foot Reflexology*. Carter sued for mail fraud.

1974 - Germany: Hanne Marquardt studied with Ingham in 1970 then publishes *Reflex Zone Therapy of the Feet*. Teaches only medical practitioners.

1975 - Europe: Heidi Masafret after working in China writes about reflexology in her book *Good Health for the Future*.

1978 - Canada: Reflexology Association of Canada (RAC) founded.

1978 - U.S.: Reflexology incorporated into rehabilation work in Piqua, Ohio.

1978 - Taiwan: Father Joseph Eugster, influenced by Masafret begins work.

1981 - U.S.: Foot Reflexology Awareness Association (FRAA) founded in Los Angeles.

1982 - U.S.: Judy Turner vs. State of Illinois - sued for practicing medicine without a license.

1982 - Taiwan: RWO-SHUR Health Institute International founded to spread Father Joseph's work.

1984 - U.S.: FRAA at the California Police Olympics.

1987 - U.S.: SVRA & FRAA work at California Police Olympics. First time two reflexology organization joined together on a project.

1989 - U.S.: First California state-wide conference of reflexologists held regardless of methodology.

1989 - U.S.: First North American conference held in Denver, Council of North American Reflexologists started.

1989 - U.S.: First research conference, sponsored by RRP and CNAR held in Piqua, Ohio.

1990 - U.S.: American Reflexology Certification Board established.

1990 - International Council of Reflexologists formed in Toronto.

1990 - U.S.: Reflexology exempt from massage laws in the states of Maine and New Mexico.

1991 - U.S.: PMS reflexology research study completed.

1992 - Australia: Global Reflexology Research Institute for Reflexologists (GRRIP) founded to gather and conduct world wide research.

1992-93 - Government funded reflexology research studies begun in Switzerland and Denmark.

1993 - U.S.: North Dakota passes first state wide reflexology law calling for establishment of a certification and registration Board.

Associations in the United States

Associated Reflexologists of Colorado
7043 West Colfax Avenue
Denver CO 80215

Foot Reflexology Awareness Association
P O Box 7622
Mission Hills CA 91346

Maine Council of Reflexologists
P O Box 969
Jefferson ME 04348

Nevada Reflexology Organization
4186 Walhaven Court
Las Vegas NV 89103

North Dakota Reflexology Association
P O Box 7
Edinburg ND 58227

Ohio Association of Reflexologists
P O Box 428725
Cincinnati OH 45242

Pennsylvania Reflexology Association
3130 Trolley Bridge Circle
Quakertown PA 18951

Reflexology Association of California
P O Box 641156
Los Angeles CA 90064

Sacramento Valley Reflexology Association
P O Box 160971
Sacramento CA 95816